NORTHERN EXPOSURES

A Canadian Perspective on Occupational Health and Environment

David Bennett

Former National Director, Health, Safety, and Environment, Canadian Labour Congress

Work, Health, and Environment Series
Series Editors: Charles Levenstein, Robert Forrant, and John Wooding

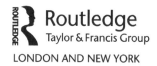

Routledge
Taylor & Francis Group

LONDON AND NEW YORK

First published 2011 by Baywood Publishing Company, Inc.

2 Park Square, Milton Park, Abingdon, Oxon OX14 4RN
711 Third Avenue, New York, NY 10017, USA

Routledge is an imprint of the Taylor & Francis Group, an informa business

First issued in paperback 2017

Library of Congress Catalog Number: 2010002770
ISBN 13: 978-0-89503-401-4 (hbk)

Library of Congress Cataloging-in-Publication Data

Bennett, David, 1943-
  Northern exposures : a Canadian perspective on occupational health and environment / David Bennett.
        p. ; cm. -- (Work, health, and environment series)
  Other title: Canadian perspective on occupational health and environment
  Includes bibliographical references and index.
  ISBN 978-0-89503-401-4 (cloth : alk. paper) 1. Industrial hygiene--Canada. 2. Environmental health--Canada. I. Title. II. Title: Canadian perspective on occupational health and environment. III. Series: Work, health, and environment series.
  [DNLM: 1. Occupational Health--Canada--Review. 2. Environmental Health--Canada--Review. 3. Public Policy--Canada--Review. WA 400 B471n 2010]
  HD7658.B46 2010
  363.110971--dc22

                                                                2010002770

ISBN 978-0-89503-401-4 (hbk)
ISBN 978-0-415-78436-8 (pbk)

In Memory of

DICK MARTIN

Secretary-Treasurer
Canadian Labour Congress

Table of Contents

Preface   vii

Acknowledgments   ix

Introduction   1

PART I. THE CANADIAN LABOR MOVEMENT

Health and Safety at the Canadian Labour Congress

Chapter 1. The Right to Know about Chemical Hazards
in Canada, 1982-2006   17

The Story of the Convergence

Chapter 2. Labour and the Environment at the Canadian Labour
Congress—The Story of the Convergence   29

PART II. PREVENTION VERSUS CONTROL: EARLY MOVES

Chapter 3. Occupational Health: A Discipline Out of Focus   39

Chapter 4. Pesticide Reduction: A Case Study from Canada   57

PART III: POLLUTION PREVENTION IN OCCUPATIONAL HEALTH AND ENVIRONMENT

Chapter 5. The Canadian Labour Congress' Pollution Prevention
Strategy   67

Chapter 6. Prevention and Transition   83

PART IV: CANCER PREVENTION

Chapter 7. Cancer Battles and the Sleep of Reason: Review 97

Books About Cancer: Pragmatic Purpose, Profound Analysis: Reviews

Chapter 8. The Politics of Cancer Revisited: Review 111
Cancer-Gate: How to Win the Losing Cancer War: Review . . . 117

Chapter 9. The Secret History of the War on Cancer: Review 125

PART V: FROM ENVIRONMENT TO SUSTAINABILITY

Sustainability: Materials Policy

Chapter 10. Industrial Materials: A Guidebook for the Future:
Review 135

The Ecology of Commerce

Chapter 11. 'Natural Capitalism's' Bold Theory: Review 141

PART VI: INTERNATIONAL REGIMES IN HEALTH, SAFETY, AND ENVIRONMENT

Chapter 12. Beware ISO 149

Chapter 13. ISO and the WTO: A Report to the International
Confederation of Free Trade Unions' Working Party on
Health, Safety, and Environment 163

Chapter 14. Health and Safety Management Systems:
Liability or Asset? 169

Index 185

Preface

In the Baywood series *Work, Health, and Environment,* the conjunction of topics is deliberate and critical. We begin at the point of production—even in the volumes that address environmental issues—because that is where things get made, workers labor, and raw materials are fashioned into products. It is also where things get stored or moved, analyzed or processed, computerized or tracked. In addition, it is where the folks who do the work are exposed to a growing litany of harmful things or are placed in harm's way. The focus on the point of production provides a framework for understanding the contradictions of the modern political economy.

Despite claims to a post-industrial society, work remains essential to all our lives. While work brings income and meaning, it also brings danger and threats to health. The point of production, where goods and services are produced, is also the source of environmental contamination and pollution. Thus, work, health, and environment are intimately linked.

Work organizations, systems of management, indeed the idea of the "market" itself, have a profound impact on the handling of hazardous materials and processes. The existence or absence of decent and safe work is a key determinant of the health of the individual and the community: what we make goes into the world, sometimes improving it, but too often threatening the environment and the lives of people across the globe.

We began this series to bring together some of the best thinking and research from academics, activists, and professionals, all of whom understand the intersection between work and health and environmental degradation, and all of whom think something should be done to improve the situation.

The works in this series stress the political and social struggles surrounding the fight for safer work and protection of the environment, and the local and global struggle for a sustainable world. The books document the horrors of cotton dust, the appalling and dangerous conditions in the oil industry, the unsafe ways in which toys and sneakers are produced, the struggles to link unions and communities to fight corporate pollution, and the dangers posed by the petrochemical industry, both here and abroad. The books speak directly about the contradictory effects of the point of production for the health of workers, community, and the environment. In all these works, the authors keep the politics front and foremost. What has emerged, as this series has grown, is a body of scholarship uniquely focused and highly integrated around themes and problems absolutely critical to our own and our children's future.

Acknowledgments

The author wishes to express warm thanks to the editors of the *Work, Health, and Environment Series*, Charles Levenstein, John Wooding, and Bob Forrant, who have been colleagues and fellow members of the health and safety movement for many years. Among American friends who have also been most helpful over the years are Ken Geiser and Joel Tickner of the Lowell Center for Sustainable Production, and Dick Clapp, the Scientific Editor of the journal *New Solutions,* as well as Mike Wright of USW, the former Chair of the International Confederation of Free Trade Unions Health, Safety and Environment Working Group.

My principal thanks are due to the members, past and present, of the Canadian Labour Congress Health, Safety and Environment Committee: Dick Martin, Hassan Yussuff, and Bill Chedore (CLC); Bob Bouchard (QFL); Andy King (USW); Larry Stoffman (UFCW); Nick DeCarlo, George Botic, Rick Coronado, Loretta Woodcock, and Cathy Walker (CAW); Brian Kohler and Keith Newman (CEP); Verna Ledger (IWA-Canada); Linda Jolley (OFL); Jeff Bennie and Donald Lafleur (CUPW); Len Bush (NUPGE); Laura Lozanski (CAUT); Denis St Jean (PSAC); Cliff Andstein, Cliff Stainsby, George Heyman, and Helga Knote (BCGEU-NUPGE); Colin Lambert and Anthony Pizzino (CUPE); John Cartwright (Carpenters/MTLC); Sarwan Boal (CFU) and Mae Burrows (United Fishers and Allied Workers Union/CAW). These individuals and their unions are largely responsible for the progress made in workplace health and safety and for the work of the Canadian labor movement in environmental protection.

I also thank Canadian environmentalists without whose leadership and example, the Canadian Labour Congress would never have become part of the mainstream environmental movement: Elizabeth May, Paul Muldoon, Steven Shrybman, Craig Bolkjovak, Susan Tanner, and the late Michelle Swenarchuk.

Special thanks are due to two individuals. Ted Schrecker has been a professional colleague for 30 years: I owe much to his vision, which is both idealistic and practical, and the cogency of his thinking. Dick Martin at the Canadian Labour Congress presided over health and safety in Canada for 2 decades and he was the driving force behind the introduction of the labor movement to the new area of environmental protection. Dick was a rare individual who was widely loved and respected, Canada's Tony Mazzocchi.

Chapter 3, Occupational Health, a Discipline Out of Focus, and Chapter 14, Health and Safety Management Systems, Liability or Asset? are reproduced with the kind permission of the editors of the *Journal of Public Health Policy.* Chapter 2, Labour and Environment at the Canadian Labour Congress, is reproduced with the kind permission and cooperation of the editors of the electronic journal, *Just Labour.* All the other chapters are articles or reviews previously published in the journal *New Solutions*.

Introduction

This book concerns the Canadian record in occupational health and environmental protection in the period from the late 1970s to the early years of the 21st century. This period coincides roughly with the years that the author spent in various health, safety, and environment positions in the national office of the Canadian Labour Congress. By the late 1970s, every Canadian province (comparable to the American states) had a workplace health and safety law and a set of regulations under the various acts of the provincial legislatures. National environmental legislation lagged somewhat behind that of the United States and it was not until 1988 that the Canadian Environmental Protection Act (CEPA) became law.

Concerning occupational health, the themes of the book rest on the development of occupational health from its foundation in legislation in the 1970s. From the point of view of environmental protection, the story begins with CEPA 1988 and continues with the relations between the labor and environmental movements from the late 1980s onwards. By a "Canadian perspective" is meant the point of view of the Canadian labor movement and, insofar as labor became a part of the mainstream environmental movement in the 1990s, that of the environmental movement too. The book is not written from a scientific point of view; but the arguments all claim to be scientifically or intellectually defensible (one of the themes in the chapters that follow is the relationship between science and health policy—occupational and environmental health). This Introduction makes clear whether the contentions in each case are made from a labor or an environmental point of view; where a personal view is put forward, it is made plain, together with the reasons for adopting that perspective.

Northern Exposures is divided into six Parts of fourteen chapters. Part I describes the part played by labor in the development of the Canadian health and safety system and its increasing involvement in the Canadian environmental movement. Part II introduces a distinction fundamental to health, safety, and environmental protection: the *prevention* of the creation of workplace and environmental pollution and the *control* or limitation of pollution once created. This is the background to the development in Part III of the concept of Pollution Prevention in occupational health and environment. The application of these ideas to the prevention of occupational and environmental cancer is covered in Part IV. Part V deals with the emergence of the concept of sustainability from its context of environmental protection. Part VI describes the role of Canadian labor in international regimes governing health, safety, and environment.

LABOR'S INVOLVEMENT IN OCCUPATIONAL HEALTH AND ENVIRONMENT

The first two chapters of this book explain how the issues of workplace health and safety and environmental protection are handled in Canada as a matter of public policy. The first chapter describes how the labor movement succeeded in establishing the Workplace Hazardous Materials Information System (WHMIS), Canada's national right-to-know law on chemical hazards.[1] The chapter begins with a description of the health and safety system in Canada. There are essentially two aspects to this system: a body of *standards*, placing a limit on the hazards of work, and a series of *rights*, establishing labor's role in the workplace governance of health and safety. Government inspectors can enforce standards and they can ensure that workers' rights are respected.

WHMIS was in many ways a "first." Up until the early 1980s, the Canadian Labour Congress's National Health and Safety Committee had loosely coordinated labor activities across the country but negotiations and consultations over health and safety standards took place at the provincial level or with the federal government in the extensive but still limited area of federal authority and jurisdiction. The result was a patchwork of *standards* and enforcement procedures, though there is quite a large degree of uniformity over workers' health and safety *rights* among the various provinces, territories, and the federal jurisdiction. WHMIS changed this system in that it produced a genuine, uniform national standard in an area where the provisions over chemical hazards were feeble, uneven, or non-existent. The project was organized by the federal government, with labor and provincial government representation; the provinces agreed to a uniform system in those parts of the WHMIS consensus that were to be implemented by the provinces rather than the federal government. For the Canadian Labour Congress (CLC), the WHMIS agreement was a tangible triumph because it secured an effective national standard in health and safety. WHMIS also enhanced the reputation and respect for the central body, both within and outside the labor movement.

Yet there was another consequence of the success of WHMIS, this time ominous, which was not evident at the time. The Canadian Chemical Producers' Association (CCPA) played a positive role both in the construction of WHMIS

---

[1] The author was the chief labor negotiator in WHMIS.

and in ensuring that it was properly implemented, a role not common for equivalent organizations in other countries, particularly in the United States. But what WHMIS did was to further entrench the CCPA in national policy-making, particularly over chemicals and environmental protection. In these areas, there are two business constituencies: the chemical *producers* and the chemical *user* companies. Measured by the volume and toxicity of chemicals in use, the latter are more important than the former, in regard to their impact on the workplace, the community and the environment. Yet it was the chemical producers who had overwhelming influence on the government's environmental policy. As will be seen, this influence came out in two main directions: the government's program for chemical assessment and for Pollution Prevention, one element of which is a reduction of the volume of toxic chemicals in use. The CCPA saw Pollution Prevention as a threat to the volume and type of chemicals that its member companies produced and did everything possible to prevent the issue becoming a matter of national policy. The user companies, who were often sympathetic to Pollution Prevention and its sub-discipline, Toxics Use Reduction (TUR), were powerless to make their influence felt; they sometimes resented the power of the CCPA. The environmental movement, including labor, was slow to recognize the politics of prevention and this was one reason why, through misguided tactics, our efforts in the 1990s failed.

The CLC became involved in environmental protection (chapter 2) in the late 1980s, at first as an offshoot of health and safety. This author was first the CLC Environmental Representative, then National Director of Health, Safety and Environment. Most of the potential environmental activists in the labor movement were novices and had a lot to learn, principally from Canadian environmentalists. The experience of the labor movement in health and safety shaped the preconceptions as to what to expect in the new area of the environment. From the start, there had been an attempt to "professionalize" the discipline of health and safety, so that workers and employers were seen as the "clients" of the professional providers: government scientists, their medical and academic advisers, company doctors, and health trainers. Instead of workers and employers creating their own regimes, with help from the professionals where needed, the agenda was to be set by the professional providers. From the perspective of the labor movement, this view of health and safety was quite perverse when it came to prevention strategies, about which most Canadian doctors knew little, since it formed no part of their outlook and training. Something parallel seemed to labor activists to be going on in the environmental movement: the first impression was that it was similarly dominated by environmental lawyers, good at figuring out legal strategies but often enough ineffectual as activists. This seemed to explain what labor believed to be a dead end in Canadian national environmental policy, at least that half that dealt with chemicals and wastes, as opposed to ecology and the natural environment.

ENVIRONMENTAL PROTECTION IN CANADA

The principal federal statute dealing with the environment is the Canadian Environmental Protection Act (CEPA) of 1988, revised in 1999. The environmentalists' contribution to the framing of CEPA was the program of sunsetting (phasing out) of toxic chemicals and pollutants from the Great Lakes. This involved a chemical classification and evaluation system, which listed chemicals slated for elimination in order of priority. There were 21 chemicals or groups of chemicals on the first priority list. So the expectation for CEPA was that there would be a similar, national program whereby there would be selected chemical "candidates" for elimination from the Canadian environment.

CEPA established the framework for the assessment and control of chemicals in use in Canada. Chemicals were graded into groups and the first group was of Priority Substances, initially 44 in number. The two government departments involved, Environment Canada and Health Canada, then performed an assessment of each chemical and produced a report. If the assessment concluded that the chemical was a threat to human health or the environment, by way of toxicity, volume used, industrial applications and risk of contamination, it was adjudged "CEPA-toxic." There was then a Strategic Options process, which looked at options for action. The chemical could then go onto a "Virtual Elimination" list, or it could be put straight on Schedule 1 of CEPA, which empowers the federal government to issue a range of measures: banning the substance, control measures, emission limits from industrial plants, limiting the amount of the substance in food, or requiring Pollution Prevention Planning (PPP). The appearance of a chemical on CEPA Schedule 1 does not guarantee significant, timely, or effective action.

Twenty years after the establishment of CEPA and the unwieldy apparatus of chemical assessment, virtually no hazardous materials have been removed from the Canadian environment. Instead of the government directly using its regulatory authority under CEPA to address a particular chemical, it has limited its action and routed its chemicals policy through the assessment procedure. Internationally, the Canadian chemical assessment process is highly regarded. The assessment process is useful in terms of the public's right to know about the dangers of toxic chemicals in the Canadian environment, but so far as control measures are concerned, it has proved to be a useless and wasteful enterprise. There are a lot of parties responsible for this state of affairs but it does seem that the environmental movement, dominated by lawyers, has been sucked into a counterproductive enterprise which is also a diversion from more effective approaches to the control of environmental pollution. There is, however, one constituency that clearly benefits from the chemical assessment procedure. The trade associations make great play of taking seriously, and participating in, the assessments; they appear to do so with the understanding that no more will be expected of them, that there will be no further burden of implementing chemical control measures.

The case of bis-phenol A (BPA), used in the resins lining food containers, is a case in point. In 2008, the government expressed its intention to put BPA on CEPA Schedule 1. There was a general celebration as Canada was the first country to move against a dangerous chemical ingested with food. At the same time, the government in the assessment process held up the review of 50 chemicals, eventually examining 18 and recommending early in 2009 that one (diethyl sulphate) be added to CEPA Schedule 1. Clearly, the assessment process continues to yield a large number of substances of great concern, only a very small number of which end up on CEPA Schedule 1—a huge administrative effort for minimal results.

In the case of BPA, the government did ban the use of the chemical in baby bottles but it could have done much more to pave the way to total elimination, beyond proposing tighter food contamination limits. The government could simply issue a requirement for both producers and users (canning companies) to produce Pollution Prevention Plans. In the case of producers, the company would be required to state what it would do to produce a less hazardous alternative or use less BPA in its production process. If the company had no plan, such a statement would comprise its plan. The BPA users, the canning companies, would be required to state their plans to use a less polluting or less toxic alternative to BPA in their products. Here, California is a model, since its moves to ban the fuel additive MTBE were accompanied by a requirement to demonstrate that substitutes are less toxic than the banned substance. The Pollution Prevention Planning requirements for BPA would increase general awareness, since public knowledge of the existence of the plans shows the pattern of food contamination and what moves, if any, are being made to phase out BPA. They would also be a signal that the government is going to do something serious about BPA, and thus give companies time to adjust, instead of merely putting a chemical on a list.

Another consequence of the assessment procedure has been to absorb energy at the expense of the new approach, Pollution Prevention and its sub-discipline, Toxics Use Reduction (TUR). These issues are dealt with in Parts II and III, chapters 3-6. The first thing that had to be done was to distinguish prevention from control. Prevention is any measure that avoids the creation or use of a polluting substance or process, while control measures (e.g., numerical emission limits or workplace exposure limits) include any limits to the effects of a pollutant once in use or created. As is shown in chapter 3, industrial hygiene practice has traditionally been weighted toward control rather than prevention, so much so that some of the foundations of the discipline need to be radically recast. Certain international instruments, such as the International Labour Organization's Convention on Occupational Health Services (1985) take workplace pollution as a "given," expecting that the workers' health will be monitored rather than that pollutants be removed "at the source," that action will be remedial rather than preventive.

In one area of prevention, Canada has made progress. Due to the efforts of environmentalists, there has been a proliferation of municipal by-laws banning or restricting the cosmetic (non-agricultural) use of chemical pesticides, when they are used on lawns, gardens, and playing fields to kill weeds and pests. Quebec has gone further: the ban on the cosmetic use of pesticides has been extended from municipalities to the entire province and, further, even the retail sale of cosmetic pesticides has been banned, a bold move that is normally a matter of federal authority. Extending elimination and use-reduction to agricultural pesticides will be much harder. Chapter 3 sketches an early attempt to frame a classification system for chemical pesticides, so that the least toxic pesticides are used, in the lowest possible quantities, an echo of the sort of system that environmentalists used in the sunsetting program for the Great Lakes. This would amount to a science-based systematization of Integrated Pest Management which (when properly construed and shorn of its abuses) is an analogue in agriculture of industrial Pollution Prevention. Despite the progress in the area of pesticide use, the shift in Canada from control to prevention has been slow and hard, as will now be seen.

POLLUTION PREVENTION

The aim of the CLC Pollution Prevention Strategy (chapter 5)[2] is to adapt the terms of the Massachusetts Toxics Use Reduction Act (1989) to Canada, with the addition that the act be specifically aimed at workplace as well as environmental pollution. One of the advantages of coming to environment as a novice is the freedom from traditional thinking and presumptions. Pollution Prevention is a case in point. The very process of the transposition was a matter not only of environmental politics but of intellectual struggle as well. The reason is arcane: the Canadian constitution. In 1981, the Canadian constitution was "repatriated" and the British North America Act of 1867 (buttressed by the Statute of Westminster of 1931) became the Constitution Act. Canada's constitution was no longer a British Act of Parliament. There were then two attempts to change the constitution, mainly to define the status of Quebec, but these failed. There were, in addition, at least three areas in which, by international standards, the Constitution Act was inadequate and which the attempts at change did not address: the foreign policy power; the undefined powers of Canada's de facto head of state, the Governor-General; and the environmental authority of the federal government. In the last case, there is no equivalent of the U.S. Interstate Commerce Clause to ensure a strong federal authority over the environment.

---

[2] For the text of the CLC Pollution Prevention Strategy, go to http://canadianlabour.ca/./sites/clc/files/shared/pollutionpreventionEn.pdf. See also Reference [1].

There was, understandably, no mention of environment in the British North America Act and this did not change with the new Constitution Act. Federal environmental authority has to be constructed from other elements of the constitution: the criminal law power; the purpose of the constitution to promote "peace, order and good government" and in areas where there is an overriding national interest at stake. The federal governmental power was in fact weakened in the Constitution Act, when authority over energy and natural resources was handed over to the provinces (off-shore oil and gas remain a federal matter). Environmentalists have feared that the formal responsibility for the three most effective federal environmental regulations, those governing mining, oil refining, and pulp and paper would be abdicated in favor of the provinces. The reality is almost as bad: absent public pressure, it is easy for the federal government to wash its hands of these areas by handing over administration and enforcement to the provinces, without any accounting or reporting requirement.

In the area of environmental protection, there is both vagueness and duplication: where there is joint responsibility under the constitution, the provinces and the federal government can shuffle off responsibility to the other party, so that little or nothing is done. But from the various heads of powers and a few cases won by the federal government, environmental lawyers have concluded that the federal government does indeed have a potentially effective environmental presence, on their widely shared presumption that a strong, unified federal authority is better than a fragmented one in securing national environmental standards. One consequence of this is that, for some environmental lawyers, a national Pollution Prevention program has to be a matter of federal legislation covering the whole country.

Pollution Prevention Planning and action are notoriously things that take place *within* workplaces, at the expense of measures implemented at the end of the waste pipe. But on this issue, the Canadian constitution is clear: issues that concern or take place within workplaces, such as industrial relations, employment standards, and health and safety, are under provincial, not federal jurisdiction; apart, that is, from federal "undertakings," workplaces covered by the Canada Labour Code. Health too is a provincial matter. Here lies a deep flaw in the whole process. In the few areas where the federal government requires Pollution Prevention Plans, it does everything possible to avoid having federal inspectors invade provincially-administered workplaces (to check on the existence and adequacy of the plans). It is also impossible to enforce a planning requirement when to do so would trespass on provincial jurisdiction. So Pollution Prevention Planning is really unenforceable and it to environmental lawyers' discredit that they have involved themselves as consultants in trying to make the impossible work.

The problem for the Canadian Labour Congress was how to reconcile a national program of Pollution Prevention with such fragmented jurisdiction. The chosen solution was that the federal government would no longer make a pretense of legislating for the whole country in the name of a national standard. Instead, the federal government would legislate only for the limited federal workplace jurisdiction. This would then become the model for the provinces to follow. The CLC devised a taxation system similar to the Massachusetts TUR fee system levied on businesses using toxic chemicals. The fees raised in a particular province would be rebated if the province implemented and enforced regulations equivalent to the federal model.

The environmentalists' objections to the CLC Pollution Prevention Strategy were manifold. The first was that the CLC's program falls short of a national standard. This is quite true but, because of the Canadian constitution, a completely genuine national standard for Pollution Prevention cannot be realized. Second, environmentalists contended that TUR does not eliminate pollution; it only reduces it. Coming from a movement that has not succeeded in any of its efforts to get toxic substances banned under CEPA, this is a highly dubious criticism. Third, TUR is soft law. It requires enforcement only at the fringes; it does not get tough with polluters. This is a valid criticism, which has appeared regularly in the pages of the journal *New Solutions,* to which the best answer is that the system needs to be based initially on cooperation and when the prevention mind-set has become entrenched, Pollution Prevention should be a regular and normal part of an enforcement regime, as is the case in other areas of activity.

In view of the skepticism of the mainline environmental movement, Pollution Prevention caught on slowly in Canada. There was yet another reason why the CLC Pollution Prevention Strategy did not take off right away: it was not well understood. Some environmentalists did not grasp what a radical change in environmental policy TUR represented. It can be the same with workers. This author conducted an exercise in an education session, which involved asking whether a series of workplace measures were a case of prevention or of control. The workers were wrong far more often than they were right.

Another example comes from the federal government. The few federal Pollution Prevention Plans mix up prevention and control, so that control measures can count as part of a plan, thus minimizing the impact and the requirements of prevention. They have also chosen industries where Pollution Prevention is likely to be the least effective: when, for instance, Pollution Prevention is applied to heavy metal smelters, it is impossible to reduce or eliminate heavy metals, as ore and product, from the smelting process except by reducing the scale of operations, something not intended.

When someone is immersed in the discipline, it is easy to lose sight of how novel the perspective of prevention really is. In the middle of this last decade, the CLC made some progress in getting a federal TUR regulation passed, so much so that the government and business looked to the CLC rather than to the mainstream environmental movement for initiative in the area. One of the challenges was to get the environmental movement to turn toward Pollution Prevention and away from the chemical assessment program, in which 20 years of work have been invested. This effort was on the whole unsuccessful and the immediate future of Pollution Prevention now lies in such provinces as Ontario, where legislation is imminent, and British Columbia—with the labor movement in the lead.

By the mid-1990s, the CLC had formed alliances with the major national and regional environmental organizations. These alliances worked on a range of issues including pesticide use reduction, regulatory policy, climate action, and sustainability. Labor's prime concern was with human health, both in the workplace and in the adjoining communities. This met with the sympathy of the environmental movement, partly because environmental health was part of its mandate and partly because human health was a useful hook in environmental campaigns. The CLC was a leader in cancer prevention campaigns, working with our allies to influence public policy and to turn the Canadian Cancer Society toward prevention; labor was a founder of Canada's leading cancer non-governmental organization, "Prevent Cancer Now!" Part IV, chapters 7, 8, and 9 (reviews) are an extension of the principles of Pollution Prevention into the health issue of cancer. These chapters expose the poverty of professional thinking on the cancer epidemic and they do so without contending or having to prove that scientists and physicians are in the pockets of big business and the pharmaceutical companies. The outlook and the philosophy of the Canadian cancer prevention movement owe much to such thinkers as Sam Epstein and Devra Davis, whose work is examined and explicated in chapters 8 and 9.

SUSTAINABILITY

When sustainable development became a public issue in the late 1980s, the first response was from environmentalists. Starting from the premise that industrial development was the prime cause of environmental degradation, they objected to any program that involved further development because it resulted in further environmental loss. This put environmentalists on a collision course with labor, since labor depends on continuous industrial development to maintain and increase employment. Environmentalists had a well-founded complaint that much sustainable development was really business as usual, citing the report (1987) of the UN World Commission on Environment and Development (the Brundtland Commission) as a case in point.

Then the debate got out of hand. Hermann Daly is regarded rightly as a founder of the concept of sustainability in his theory of steady-state economics, which does not depend on continuous growth, a breach of the first environmental commandment. He reluctantly conceded that there would have to be some development in the less industrialized countries, which some environmentalists took as evidence that Daly was not really a true believer in zero growth. The debate should really have been about the type and extent of industrial change needed to achieve sustainability, such as powering African villages with solar instead of large hydro-electric dams and the electrical grid. More generally, sustainable development means a transition to alternative energy sources and sustainable industrial production: the "steady state" is reached when the major transitions to sustainability have been achieved. The challenge for the labor movement is how to do this while maintaining union membership, levels of employment and income, and healthy workplaces. So labor developed the programs of Green Job Creation[3] and Just Transition for Workers During Environmental Change,[4] (chapters 2 and 6).

At its extreme, the debate was over two arguments which really led nowhere. First, some environmentalists said that the increasingly heavy use of fossil fuels (what the late John Updike called "using up the environment") would lead to the end of life on earth. They cited the Second Law of Thermodynamics, which says that a closed system with different energy levels within it, will end up with a uniform level of energy, a state of quiescence or entropy. The trouble is that the earth is not a closed system; it has a constant input of free energy in the form of the sun. This means that the appeal to the Second Law is not pertinent. Hence, the fatuous criticisms of solar energy systems that they only manage to harness a low percentage of the available energy.

Second, some environmentalists came to see sustainable development as an all-or-nothing concept: an activity is either sustainable or it is not. Any human activity which involved any amount of degradation of the environment was not sustainable; true sustainability could only be achieved with a human terrestrial population of around 200,000. The most obvious answer is to develop an index of sustainability in which activities are graded according to criteria and placed on a scale with minimum sustainability at one end and maximum sustainability at the other.

There is a huge amount of literature on sustainable energy policy but almost none on materials policy, with the major exception of the issues covered in chapter 10 (a review). There was one aspect of sustainable development in which environmentalists were undoubtedly correct. This was the abuse of the term, usually by businesspeople, to show that their activities really were sustainable or that alternative strategies were not so, often because they were not cost-effective. Chapter 11 (review) on Natural Capitalism is a useful corrective to this view. Yet, in all, it is understandable that in view of the abuses of the concept, environmentalists now prefer to talk of sustainability rather than sustainable development.

---

[3] For the CLC Green Job Creation Strategy, go to http:canadianlabour.ca/en/green_job_creation_paper

[4] For the CLC Policy Statement on Just Transition, go to canadianlabour.ca/sites/clc/files/updir/justransen.pdf

HEALTH, ENVIRONMENT, AND GLOBALIZATION

In the early 1980s, the CLC became a leading member of the Health, Safety and Environment Working Group of the International Confederation of Free Trade Unions (ICFTU, now the ITUC). One of the main functions of the ICFTU was to serve as a constituent and consulting member of the International Labour Organization (ILO). The role of the ILO in workplace health and safety is explained in Part VI, chapters 12, 13, and 14. Labor's involvement with the ICFTU and, through it, the ILO coincided with the globalization of the world economy.

The concept of globalization is plagued by a wide misunderstanding of its meaning and the extent of its actualization in the world. In its proper sense, globalization means the ability of businesses to move money, labor, and goods throughout the world, without hindrance from national boundaries and without restriction, for instance in the form of financial, environmental, or labor laws. This process is facilitated by free trade agreements, such as the World Trade Organization (WTO) Agreement and the North American Free Trade Agreement (NAFTA), both dating from 1994. These agreements deal with national economies, ostensibly promoting free trade between nations. In practice, extensive national provisions for tariffs and subsidies were legitimized in the agreements, so that trade was "free" for large corporations in highly industrialized countries with corresponding detriments for the less developed.

One of the misconceptions about the WTO Agreement and NAFTA is that they deal only with economic, trade, and financial matters. In reality, the social provisions of the agreements are as important as the economic in pursuing the globalization agenda and they have a direct impact on health, safety, and environment. This is explained in chapters 12 and 13.[5] In particular, what the agreements try to do is to subordinate national standards in such areas as environmental protection, food safety, healthcare provisions, product safety, workplace health and safety, inspection departments and chemicals policy to international regimes and standardization. This has had two consequences. One is that the international rules are invariably weaker and less comprehensive than national ones. Another is that the way in which social movements have made progress, both within countries and internationally, is by winning practices locally, which then become enshrined in laws covering the whole country, thus moving from the local to the national. These can then be advanced as national precedents for international norms. The health and safety conventions of the ILO are a case in point. The provisions of free trade agreements make this progress much more difficult: national regulations are subordinate to international provisions and countries must follow international standards wherever this is feasible. The aim is

---

[5] For critiques of free trade agreements, see also References [2, 3].

international harmonization. The main source of these standards is the International Organization for Standardization (ISO), which is discussed in chapter 12.

In some areas, the interests of labor have clashed directly with those of business in the international organizations. ISO, having produced a comprehensive set of standards for (product) Quality Management, then Environmental Management, attempted to move into the area of workplace health and safety management. The ILO forestalled this move by producing its own Guidelines on Health and Safety Management Systems (2001), giving rise to an argument as to whether or not the guideline was WTO-compliant. The development of the ILO standard is discussed in chapter 14. What labor hoped was that national health and safety management standards (of which there were already several) would be influenced by the ILO model rather than by the management models in the ISO environmental standards. In Canada, labor succeeded with the Canadian Standards Association Health and Safety Management Systems Standard (Z1000), which is, it is believed, the only national standard to include compliance with collective agreements in workplace audits of the standard.

In both NAFTA and the WTO Agreement, there is a requirement, broadly, that any national standard must be the product of a risk assessment. This issue too is dealt with in chapters 13 and 14.[6] Much of the CLC's work, both nationally and internationally, was dedicated to preventing risk assessment from becoming the driving force of public health policy in framing standards and in policy areas such as toxic chemicals, pesticides, and food safety. The premise was that, while risk assessment in itself is a respectable technique, its application in such areas as chemical safety and Maximum Residue Limits (MRLs) for pesticides will always systematically underrate the hazards and risks to human health. The general provision of free trade agreements is that policies over the results of risk assessment must be commensurate with the risk, no more. The effect is that national health policies and international standards, the preferred instrument of national policy, will always be feeble at best.

Any policies, such as Pollution Prevention and (properly interpreted) Integrated Pest Management (IPM), which are based on hazard rather than risk assessment, are always liable to succumb to the requirements of free trade agreements. Thus, Quebec's bold decision to ban the sale of cosmetic pesticides could well be subject to a NAFTA challenge. There is a project called the Globally Harmonized System for Chemical Classification and Labeling (GHS), which is intended to produce a uniform international standard for the right to know about chemical hazards (in the name, incidentally, of free trade). There are attempts to turn the GHS into a risk-based system, so that the only information available will be about significant risks, not the hazards of chemicals based on their intrinsic toxicity.

[6]For risk assessment, see References [2, 4, 5].

THE CANADIAN RECORD IN OCCUPATIONAL
HEALTH AND ENVIRONMENT

Northern Exposures covers the last quarter of the 21th century onwards, by which time Canada had enacted its health and safety laws and regulations. For the labor movement, this was a success story. The movement was effective in the first steps toward addressing systematically the hazards of work; it fell behind somewhat in the attempts to have regulations keep up with the emergence of new workplace hazards and to maintain an effective government enforcement system. The threats to these achievements are several, of which globalization is only one. Some unions such as the ITUC have abolished their health and safety services for members or constituents; others have downgraded their importance in the work of the union. Young activists no longer gravitate toward health and safety, as they did in the 1970s. In Canada, one particular threat is subordinating health and safety (sometimes called "prevention") to the Workers' Compensation system. Education and enforcement activities are then geared only to those identified by workers' compensation claims. Since the health hazards of work are far greater than those of physical injury (previously called "accidents") and since most workplace health detriments such as occupational cancer go uncompensated, the result will be essentially to take workplace health off the public agenda.

Similarly, the labor movement was hugely successful in building environmental coalitions and impacting public policy in such areas as chemical management (a misnomer, as Part VI shows), climate action, and the framework of regulation. This involved a change in attitude and outlook on the part of both labor and the environmental movement. Environmental issues recede in importance whenever jobs and the general economy are under threat. But the long-term trend is unmistakable; we need more environmentalism in labor, not less. One possibility for the future is to make environmental health the fount of labor policy, of which occupational health is an integral part. While one first reaction would be to suggest that this is not really labor's true agenda, another would be that labor needs environmentalists to restore workplace health to a prime concern. This is exactly what the Canadian Labour Congress tried to do with Pollution Prevention and Toxics Use Reduction.

REFERENCES

1. D. Bennett, *Benefits of Pollution Prevention and Cleaner Production Technologies* in the *ILO Encyclopedia of Occupational Health and Safety,* Geneva, 1996 edition.
2. D. Bennett, Harmonization and Risk Assessment in the North American Free Trade Agreement, in *Growth, Trade and Environment Values,* T. Schrecker and J. Dalgleish (eds.), Westminister Institute for Ethics and Human Values, London, Ontario, Chapter 6, 1994.
3. D. Bennett, The Process of Harmonization Under NAFTA, reprinted in *New Solutions,* 6:1, pp. 91-95, 1995.

4. Leading critiques of risk assessment are Ginsburg, R.: "Quantitative Risk Assessment and the Illusion of Safety," *New Solutions, 3*:2, Winter 1993; O'Brien, M., *Making Better Environmental Decisions, An Alternative to Risk Assessment, Part I, What Is Wrong With Risk Assessment?* MIT, Cambridge, 2000; and "Trading Away Public Health: WTO Obstacles to Effective Toxics Controls," *Journal of Public Health Policy, 21*:3, 2000.
5. D. Bennett, Risk Assessment as a Regulatory Device, in *Regulatory Efficiency and the Role of Risk Assessment,* Z. M. Mehta (ed.), Queen's University Press, Kingston, Ontario, 1995.

PART I

The Canadian Labor Movement

CHAPTER 1

The Right to Know About Chemical Hazards in Canada, 1982-2006

Traditionally in Canada, there are three health and safety rights: the right to participate (joint workplace health and safety committees); the right to refuse unsafe and unhealthy work; and the right to know about workplace hazards. By the end of the 1970s, the right to know had been established in law across Canada, but it was not enough to cover workplace chemical hazards in particular. The Workplace Hazardous Materials Information System (WHMIS) was a project set up by the Canadian federal government in 1982 to address the issue. This chapter tells the story of how labor got the progressive WHMIS agreement(1985) and how the agreement has been implemented in the following years.

By 1980, all of the Canadian provinces and territories had health and safety legislation and regulations. So too did the federal government which has jurisdiction over the federal public sector and selected private industries, an extensive authority but far less than that of the Occupational Safety and Health Administration (OSHA) in the United States. In Canada, statute law establishes a framework for the regulations and incorporates provisions for the enforcement of health and safety law. Some sections cover substantive issues, such as the rules for the establishment of joint worker-management health and safety committees in the workplace and the complex procedures over refusals to do unsafe or unhealthy work.

The regulations under the law, which are easier to institute, cover essentially two things: *standards,* which set limits on the hazards of work, and *rights,* such as the right to refuse, the right to know, and the right to a joint committee in the workplace. There is some variation in the details of these rights in Canadian law across the country but the drift is similar. Over standards, the number of regulations and their content indicates much more variation, as does their quality, ranging from vague performance requirements to highly specific provisions. The greatest variation is over enforcement. The easiest way to deregulate is simply to stop enforcing the law.

The first law in the new era of health and safety was that of Saskatchewan in 1972, two years after the Occupational Safety and Health (OSH) Act in the U.S. and two years before the Health and Safety at Work Act in the UK. The Saskatchewan law came about under the influence of Bob Sass, Associate Deputy Minister of Labour, and it is largely to him that we owe the particular evolution of health and safety in Canada. Not only did the Saskatchewan law set the tone of Canadian legislation but its precepts found their way into the generic health and safety convention of the International Labour Organization (ILO), No. 155 in 1981. The Saskatchewan law was heavy on worker participation in health and safety and the articulation of three health and safety rights: the right to participate in the form of joint workplace committees; the right to refuse unsafe or unhealthy work; and the right to know—information, education and training from the employer. It needs to be pointed out that the language of rights rarely appears in the Canadian legislation, only references to the functions and powers of workers and their unions. The emphasis placed by labor on rights may in one respect be counter-productive, because it has often occurred at the expense of health and safety standards in the workplace. You can have plenty of rights in a dangerous workplace with no standards worth the name.

Of these three rights, the right to refuse was a peculiarly North American phenomenon, which grew out of the statutory prohibition on strikes during the lifetime of a collective agreement, which is the case in Canadian law though not, ironically, in Saskatchewan in the 1970s. Hence, the complexities and limitations on the right to refuse, to ensure that a refusal is not really a strike. When I taught shop stewards in the UK in the late 1970s, I tried to interest them in a statutory right to refuse. They shrugged their shoulders and said "we do it anyway." This was at a time when the British industrial relations system was unstructured and liberal. In the particular context of health and safety, the right to know came (it seems) from two sources: as one of the tools to enable joint committees and worker representatives to do their job and information that has to be provided by the employer in order to make their worker training obligations effective.

Why was the right to know not good enough to cover chemical hazards in the workplace? The reason is that much of the information on chemical hazards does not emanate from the employer but from the supplier—the manufacturer, distributor, or importer—of the chemical product. Unless information is provided to workers and employers by chemical suppliers, no systematic knowledge of chemical hazards is possible. There was certainly a right-to-know movement in both Canada and the U.S. in the 1970s; the way it was realized in the 1980s was due to the relationship between the structure of industrial society and the requirements of health and safety law.

THE WORKPLACE HAZARDOUS INFORMATION SYSTEM (WHMIS)

The WHMIS project was set up in August 1982, comprising a Steering Committee and several working groups. The project was tripartite, which reflected both Canadian practice and the structure and operating procedure of the ILO since it was established in 1919. In theory, the three parties—labor, business, and government—were equal. Though the Steering Committee had of course no executive authority, labor and business expected that consensus proposals would be adopted by government as a package, not cherry-picked or shelved. Both of these suppositions, of the equality of the parties and the expectations of the non-government representatives, were in practice qualified and there were complexities within the three constituencies which belied the simple tripartite structure of the project.

First, the government group. Not only were there representatives of provincial governments on the Steering Committee but several federal government ministries were represented, of which the principals were Labour Canada, the Department of Consumer and Corporate Affairs, and Health and Welfare Canada. Of these, only Labour Canada had any commitment to tripartite consultations; Consumer and Corporate Affairs was inexperienced and Health Canada was in practice hostile. Health Canada's personnel thought that they alone had the authority and the professional expertise to determine matters of national health and they were as much of a nuisance to Labour Canada as they were to the labor representatives on the project. One result was that Health Canada produced a list of WHMIS hazard criteria early in the project, a key part of WHMIS which decided which products came under the system and which were excluded. They refused to modify these criteria, so the labor group produced a further criterion for inclusion in WHMIS, namely whether a chemical ingredient in a product was on an Ingredient Disclosure List.

Then there were the government lawyers, who had their own ideas of where the dividing line between federal and provincial authority ought to be drawn and how the provisions in the two segments should be framed. We had endless trouble with the lawyers in the implementation phase of WHMIS, because they failed to grasp that tripartite discussions made different demands on government legislators than did those emanating from elected representatives and government officials. We were saved from impasse and breakdown at one phase by counsel in the Justice Department, Maurice Rosenberg, who had a good grasp of tripartism and had the imagination to implement what the parties wanted, not what government lawyers habitually did. He is now Deputy Minister (senior bureaucrat) in the federal Department of Health.

There were also tensions within the business group. For instance, the Canadian Chemical Producers' Association (CCPA) represented the chemical suppliers while the Canadian Manufacturers' Association (CMA) represented the workplace employers. The former were wary of disclosing what they regarded as confidential business information while the latter needed information in order to fulfill their legal duties. Thus the concerns of the CMA reflected those of labor, though for different reasons. Yet one of the main driving forces for WHMIS, was Jean Belanger, the President of the CCPA. He realized that the chemical industry had a bad public reputation and was determined to change that image, not as is usual by public relations and false propaganda but by action. Belanger, a former federal bureaucrat, was also influential at the highest levels of government. While the labor group did a good job in framing, then implementing, WHMIS, the fact remains that business pressure was important in achieving the end result.

There was also tension between big and small business. Small business balked at some of the disclosure provisions which it found costly to implement, complaining that the broad backs of corporate business were far better able to carry WHMIS than small producers, of which about a hundred belonged to the relevant trade associations. They thought they had been sold out by big business. It fell to Doug Cook, Environmental Control Manager of Imperial Oil (Exxon in Canada), to try to claw back in informal discussions what had been conceded in the formal negotiations. He did not succeed.

Outside of labor, there were a number of individuals who were instrumental in getting a good agreement and having it implemented: Belanger, Cook, Gordon Lloyd (Manager of the Technical Department of the CMA), Mark Daniels (federal Deputy Minister of Labour), and Brian Connell (Director of Health and Safety Services at the New Brunswick Occupational Health and Safety Commission, a tripartite organization).

Labor, business, and government each had three members on the WHMIS Steering Committee. The labor members were the Canadian Labour Congress (CLC) Executive Vice-President Richard Mercier, Robert Bouchard (Health and Safety Director at the Quebec Federation of Labour), and myself as CLC National Representative, Workplace Health and Safety. I attended my first WHMIS Steering Committee meeting in February 1983, before I was appointed health and safety rep. Though there had been provision for health and safety at the CLC since 1962, I was the first national rep, paid by the Congress rather than some form of government grant. As is usual with central labor bodies, there was tension between the staff of the central body and the representatives of the affiliated unions. WHMIS was the first attempt by the CLC to negotiate a national standard in workplace health and safety and some of the affiliated union reps were reluctant to have the CLC negotiate on behalf of workers who came under provincial labor jurisdiction.

That the project was kept on the rails was due to two individuals in particular. One was Robert Bouchard whose adroitness and diplomacy ensured that provincial rights would not compromise a national project. He even negotiated many of the trade secret provisions of WHMIS, which were essentially a federal matter to which the provinces were enjoined to subscribe. The other was Linda Jolley, a consultant to the CLC who later became Health and Safety Director at the Federation of Labour in Ontario, where she had played a central part in framing the province's health and safety legislation (1976). Her knowledge of health and safety, both technical and political, was enormous; without her, we would not have been able to put forward and evaluate the proposals that came under discussion.

One of the first things the labor group did was to produce a Submission in May 1983. It covered all the WHMIS issues, including the format and disclosure provisions for chemical data sheets (MSDS). We argued that WHMIS should incorporate a chemical testing regime for the chemicals covered and that there should be no protection for trade secrets. Of these, both were failures, though the trade secret provisions of WHMIS were in the event strict and, arguably, not over-protective of business interests. In general, we knew what we wanted but simply did not know what to expect—the attitude of the other two parties, what would be easy and what would be difficult, and what political maneuvering would be required in view of the complexities of the project and the various interests involved. WHMIS was new, both as an area of consultation and in the idea of a national health and safety standard.

An example concerned the possible scope of trade secret protection. We early made a distinction between the disclosure of chemical identities (chemical names of the ingredients of a product) and "hazard information" which was information, including toxicity data, *about* the chemicals named. Before we got into serious discussions about trade secrets at the Steering Committee, Linda Jolley and I went to a meeting at the CCPA. We asked what trade secret provisions would, in the business view, apply to hazard information. Imagine our surprise when Dr. David Dawes of DuPont paused, then said "none at all." This happened at a time when "proprietary data" for pesticides was claimed as both confidential and proprietary (that is, competitors could not submit data originally generated by another manufacturer) so our surprise was understandable. Now the idea that hazard information is non-confidential is commonplace, at least for industrial chemicals, if not for food, drugs, pesticides, and environmental contaminants.

THE WHMIS AGREEMENT

From the beginning, WHMIS was envisaged as a triad: a label, a data sheet, and a worker education program. In the final agreement, the label was for immediate safe handling of the chemical product and there was a link on the label to the data sheet, which was a further elaboration of hazard information. The supplier is obliged to disclose on the data sheet, hazard information in his possession or which he ought reasonably to be aware of. The worker education program was the final element of the WHMIS triad and it was later embodied in a model workplace regulation. This model would be adopted by all the provincial and territorial health and safety authorities as well as the federal workplace jurisdiction under Part IV of the Canada Labour Code (now renumbered as Part II). The model regulation also contained requirements for the labeling in the workplace of pipes, piping system and valves, and additionally, rules about the accessibility to workers of data sheets.

The rules over labels, data sheets and trade secrets are a federal responsibility. Thus WHMIS was a dovetailing of federal and provincial responsibilities, a relatively rare and successful example of what is called in Canada "cooperative federalism." The chemical names of the hazardous ingredients of a product do not appear on the label, a weakness in WHMIS. A sample model data sheet was appended to the WHMIS Steering Committee Report but it was an illustration only, not part of the WHMIS Agreement. When the requirements for data sheets came out, they did in fact include the categories and sub-categories of information according to the WHMIS model. Suppliers are allowed to enter "not known" or "not applicable" in the hazard information categories but not for the hazardous ingredients (chemical identities), nor items that are required under other legislation, such as the Lethal Dose (LD) and Lethal Concentration (LC) figures. Disclosure of hazard information is reinforced by the "ought reasonably to be aware of" rule. When the regulations appeared, they contained an important but rarely used provision: on request, a supplier must disclose the sources of the information that appears on the data sheet, short of disclosing items legally confirmed as a trade secret (WHMIS Agreement, Sec 30; Controlled Products Regulation under the Hazardous Products Act, Section 31).

INGREDIENT DISCLOSURE AND TRADE SECRETS

The key sections of the data sheet are the Hazardous Ingredients and Toxicological Properties. Acting on advice from Franklin Mirer of the United Auto Workers (UAW), Linda Jolley and I put forward four criteria for disclosure on the data sheet of the chemical names of the hazardous ingredients:

- an ingredient that meets one or more of the WHMIS hazard criteria;
- an ingredient of which nothing is known about its toxicological properties;
- an ingredient which is on the WHMIS Ingredient Disclosure List; and
- an ingredient which the supplier has any reason to believe may be hazardous.

With minor qualifications, these criteria were accepted: an ingredient that meets one or more of these criteria must be disclosed. The data sheet also lists the portion of the ingredient in the mixture or formulation. So as not to invite too many trade secret claims, percentage ranges are permitted. When the time came, we ensured that these four crucial criteria were embodied in legislation, not in regulation, making them more difficult for a hostile government to change. This move does, admittedly, cut both ways, since updating a provision in statute law is as difficult as deregulation.

The hardest issue was trade secrets, bringing discussions to a virtual halt early in 1984. Then labor proposed a formula: we will accept genuine trade secrets if business agrees to a maximum disclosure of information that is compatible with preservation of the trade secret. This was unanimously adopted by the Steering Committee. It was an eerie feeling: an item in the middle of a routine meeting which passed with little discussion but which meant that we would indeed get WHMIS as a good, though imperfect agreement.

Hammering out the details of a trade secret mechanism was more difficult. Trade secrets could be claimed only over the identity of ingredients, over information that would reveal a trade secret or the portion of the ingredient in a product. It was agreed that there should be a "third-party screening agency" (in practice a government body) to make a determination of trade secrecy. The determination would also include a decision as to whether the hazard information on a data sheet was commensurate with the identity of the chemical concealed as a trade secret. Decisions could be appealed by any interested party to an Arbitration Panel comprising representatives each of labor, business, and government and there would be a provision for Judicial Review. In the end, or at the beginning if there were no appeal, the trade secret would be confirmed and noted as such on the data sheet or, if denied, the supplier would have to alter the data sheet. The Arbitration Panel could also order the supplier to enter into confidentiality agreements with relevant interested parties, that is, disclosure of chemical identities on a confidential basis to workers and employers.

There was agreement as to the criteria for trade secrecy. The criteria excluded the ability to identify the trade secret through reverse engineering, that is, chemical analysis. This was understandable since with enough effort and equipment, it is possible to crack most unknown ingredients in an industrial chemical product. Trade secrets are a matter of degree, reflecting business secrecy about operations, not something perpetually shrouded in mystery.

The impasse over trade secrets led the government representatives to recommend the Canadian adoption of the draft OSHA Hazard Communication Rule. It was rejected by labor on the grounds, obvious enough, that the trade secret provisions of the Rule were unsatisfactory, permitting trade secrecy merely by assertion (trade secrets are what business says they are) with only confidentiality agreements as a solution. One criticism of WHMIS is that unless there is an arbitration (which proved to be rare events) confidentiality agreements are difficult to obtain: once there is a trade secret, it is hard for any interested party to get access to the trade secret item.

Another criticism of WHMIS is that there is a trade secret mechanism at all. In the original Saskatchewan legislation, for example, there was no protection of business confidentiality. This is to miss the point: health and safety legislation places obligations on employers, not essentially on suppliers. Much WHMIS information is something to which employers would not otherwise have had access. There are plenty of arguments against trade secrecy and labor made them: few things are really secret and trade secrecy is always a limit on the right to know. By conceding trade secrecy, we were able to make gains elsewhere: a strong consensus that would ensure the implementation of WHMIS across the country and some strong provisions over ingredient disclosure. It is easy to be pure and ineffectual.

Further, in the absence of an agreement on trade secrets, the government would simply have introduced a provision for handling confidential business information. In this case, labor would have been shut out of the process, which would have amounted to little more than a confirmation by the government of whatever business considered confidential.

IMPLEMENTATION AND ENFORCEMENT

There are three sets of legislation for WHMIS:

1. Changes to the federal Hazardous Products Act and Regulations which set the rules for labels and data sheets and which implement the Ingredient Disclosure List.
2. A new Hazardous Materials Information Review Act to institute the trade secret provisions and to set up a Hazardous Materials Information Review Commission (HMIRC), with a tripartite Council of Governors. The government group on the Council includes representatives of provincial and territorial governments. The Commission fulfills the role of the "screening agency" recommended in the WHMIS Agreement.
3. The implementation of the model WHMIS workplace regulation in the twelve health and safety jurisdictions in Canada.

After a hiatus which was really a pause for breath, labor and business embarked on a road show to persuade governments to adopt WHMIS. There was an informal understanding that business would not advocate less than the WHMIS Agreement and labor would not advocate more, a move that proved successful. There are some small variations in a few of the provincial regulations and one or two do contain provisions that go outside, rather than beyond, WHMIS.

Promotion of the WHMIS Agreement by labor and business was not, however, the main reason why it was implemented. When the WHMIS Agreement was published in April 1985, I asked Jim Black, the Director of Product Safety at Consumer and Corporate Affairs Canada, how long it would take to implement WHMIS, he replied "about ten years," par for the course but entirely unacceptable. When the federal government dragged its feet, more out of bureaucratic inertia than hostility, Ontario declared that unless there was prompt action, the province would go it alone over the right to know, the very thing that WHMIS was designed to avoid.

What followed was industrial action. There were Canadian Auto Workers (CAW) mass work refusals over the right to know and conditions of work at the Macdonnell Douglas and DeHavilland aircraft plants (and other CAW workplaces) in Toronto, Ontario, in 1986 and 1987. These mass work refusals shut down the plants for weeks. Due to the introduction of chemicals used in composite materials, new to aircraft production, workers had been getting respiratory problems and rashes. They wanted to know what they were using and didn't want to wait decades to find out that these new chemicals had long-term effects on their health, such as cancer. The work refusals were upheld by the Ontario Ministry of Labour. The companies were required to label containers, provide material safety data sheets, and pay for education and training of the work force. The courses were developed by the union and delivered by union instructors. Front page stories in newspapers across the country ensured that people throughout Canada knew about this militant action and the reasons for it. The implementation of WHMIS was a direct result of industrial action. The federal legislation for WHMIS was passed by parliament in 1987. The WHMIS legislation and regulations came into effect in October 1988, the year after the mass work refusals and the whole system, comprising the three legislated elements above, came fully into force in 1989.

Because of labor pressure, the training, communication and labeling provisions in the workplace have been implemented quite well. There is a high degree of compliance with the labeling provisions in the Hazardous Products Act. "WHMIS Training" has become an industry. The rules over data sheets have been less successful, partly because many chemical suppliers are American and subject to a different set of rules. Very many of the hundred thousand data sheets are out of compliance, ranging from minor formatting breaches, mistakes, and omissions to major abuses of the right to know. Almost all the enforcement of the data sheet rules by government inspectors of workplaces concern the absence of data sheets or their inaccessibility to workers. There is almost no quality control.

The only real enforcement of the data sheet rules comes through the trade secret mechanism and the submission of claims to the HMIRC, which have run from 69 to 245 per year in the period 1998 to 2004. Much to business's chagrin, the HMIRC lays down requirements for the whole data sheet, not just those parts relating to the trade secret claim. The two categories of Ingredient Disclosure and Toxicological Properties are the most crucial in regard to trade secret claims, comprising 54.2% of all MSDS violations in a total of twelve categories. Labor has insisted on compliance with all aspects of the data sheet rules, not just those concerning trade secrets, for the simple reason that claims submitted to the HMIRC are really the sole source of quality control and WHMIS enforcement.

Consider the problem. Chemical pesticides were among the products excluded from WHMIS in the Hazardous Products Act, the intention being either to remove the exclusions or bring the exclusions up to WHMIS standards. Only now is a data sheet requirement for chemical pesticides being introduced. There are some seven thousand pesticides registered in Canada, all of which have gone through a thorough (though permissive) process in which the government has access to all of the information summarized on the pesticide data sheet. Conformity is thus easy to detect and monitor.

Since, however, there is no comprehensive chemical testing program for industrial chemicals already in use ("existing substances"), all enforcement has to be after data sheets have been issued. For chemicals new to the market, it would be possible to compare the information on a "new" chemical ingredient with the information submitted to government as part of the Notification of New Substances Regulations. But for existing substances, the problem is much greater and less certain, since it is hard to get suppliers to come clean about their test data and other information which is in their possession and not on publicly accessible databases.

It is still possible to make progress, for example, by setting up a government certification system for data sheets over which there are no trade secret issues at stake. The certification procedure would only apply to the Ingredient Disclosure and Toxicological Properties sections of the data sheet. Certification would not exempt suppliers from their compliance obligations, since certification is not a guarantee that all relevant information has been divulged. What certification would do is to provide some assurance to workers and employers that the key sections of the data sheet are a reliable guide to the necessary prevention and control measures in the workplace.

For years, the labor movement used data sheets only for legitimate yet routine purposes such as safe handling of hazardous materials and proper control measures. With the emergence of campaigns against toxic substances such as Cancer Prevention Coalitions in the 1990s, things changed. Workers began to use data sheets as the starting point for identifying candidates for elimination from the workplace and the identification of less hazardous substitutes. Thus WHMIS has had a twofold benefit: it is a tool for improving safety and it is the first link in a chain leading to the detoxification of the workplace.

WHMIS is also a basis for the community right to know, since data sheets could also be made available to the public and to municipal authorities. But we need more than WHMIS data sheets for the community right to know, such as publicly known inventories of chemicals used in workplaces and reporting on chemical use. As Rich Whate, a Health Promotion Consultant in the Toronto Public Health Department said, "WHMIS is good, but not good enough."

ACKNOWLEDGMENTS

The author extends warm thanks to Cathy Walker, retired Director of Health, Safety and Environment at the Canadian Auto Workers, for supplying the details of the CAW industrial action in the 1980s and for her comments on an earlier draft of the article.

SOURCES

Final Report of the Workplace Hazardous Information Steering Committee to the Deputy Minister of Labour Canada, April 1985, Labour Canada Catalogue No. L46-1568/85E.

A Submission to the Steering Committee of the Hazardous Materials Information System by the Canadian Labour Congress, May 1983.

Health and Safety at Work, Report of the Committee 1970-72, Chairman Lord Robens, London, HMSO, July 1972.

Health and Safety at Work Act, UK, 1974.

Hazardous Product Act (1985); Controlled Products Regulations and the Ingredient Disclosure List Regulation (1988).

Hazardous Materials Information Review Act (1985) and the Regulations (1985), amended 2002.

Hazardous Materials Information Review Commission, Annual Report, 2004-2005. Canada Labour Code, Part II, Health and Safety, and Regulations.

CHAPTER 2

Labour and the Environment at the Canadian Labour Congress— The Story of the Convergence

GETTING INTO HEALTH AND SAFETY IN CANADA

When I came to Canada from the United Kingdom in 1980, the labor movement was expanding, both in numbers and in nature. One such change was a huge increase in union staff and the ratio of staff to rank-and-file members. With the rise of political and social action, union leaders found that they needed far more personnel than organizing and service reps. They needed researchers, educators and staff to coordinate new and (then) relatively specialized functions such as health and safety, women's issues, human rights, social justice and political action. This often meant going outside the labor movement to recruit experienced or qualified people.

These moves were not always welcomed by labor, from the grass roots to the top leadership. Often, such outsiders were categorized as "academics," alienated from the true union fraternity and not really a part of the movement. As someone who got a university degree before having to work for a living, I counted as an academic. We were members of the clique of "union bureaucrats," so despised by the real academics, whose own place in the established social order was usually far more entrenched than we pseudo-academics. Now that about half of union members have some tertiary education and the specialized functions are part of the mainstream, we hear far less about academics, except from the true academics, for whom the labor movement is never what they want it to be.

Coming from England, there were many things to learn. Not least the Canadian industrial relations system, which was very different from that of the British Isles. In Britain, the industrial relations system was informal with collective agreements that were not legally binding, little arbitration, few limitations on who could be organized and few restrictions on the right to strike. In Canada, by contrast, governments had imposed a framework on industrial relations with, of course, legally binding collective agreements, restrictions on organizing and industrial action, and draconian penalties for both unions and members who broke the rules.

Next, there was the whole culture of trade unionism—again rather different from the British. Even by British standards, my own union, the Fire Brigades' Union (FBU), was unusual. It had about 33,000 members. These included the retained (part-time) firefighters, the British equivalent of Canadian volunteers. The union also included some of the senior fire officers. So you had situations where officers had a disciplinary function, yet their policies could be criticized to their face in a union meeting. "Better have them in the tent pissing out, than outside pissing in."

The biggest difference was that the firefighters' union had no paid staff, only elected officers, a few secretaries, and a part-time journalist to edit the union magazine. All the work was done by the grass roots rank-and-file and the elected union officers, regional and national, most of whom were also full-time firefighters. This direct democracy is easier to realize in a small union than in a large one. Though I detested the Stalinist leadership, the union organization on the fire stations was superb. The shop stewards held regular meetings to discuss issues and the tenor of life on the watches (shifts). They in turn reported to the branch (fire station) union officers. Union meetings were held on the fire stations and were exceptionally well-attended, bearing in mind that there was a captive audience of the firefighters on duty and it was not a great inconvenience for the day shift to stay at the workplace for the evening union meeting. I have no doubt that this union organization was a product of the Communist politics of the 1930s.

If the FBU was unusual in Britain, it was even more so when compared to Canada. One big difference was the ratio of staff to members, which was much higher in Canada. This was partly due to the need for servicing in a highly structured and legally-mandated industrial relations system and partly because of the need for specialized union services, mentioned earlier. On emigrating to Canada, I had to learn a whole new union culture, as well as a wholly different system of industrial relations and labor standards.

Finally, there was health and safety. In this area, there was less difference between Canada and Britain, since both had health and safety laws, regulations and codes of practice. In the United States, the great promoters of health and safety were the COSH Committees (Committees on Occupational Safety and Health), community organizations with a greater or smaller number of union rank-and-file members. They were pressure groups which existed because of the union leadership's failure to take up health and safety. There was less of a need for COSH groups in Canada, but health and safety activists still had the reputation as shit-disturbers, bent on making trouble both for and within unions. One former Canadian Labour Congress (CLC) President was reluctant to hire a health and safety staff representative on the curious grounds that health and safety was a workplace issue. So there was no need for a national presence. I became the CLC Health and Safety representative in 1983, transferring from the Education Department.

By this time, all of the provinces and territories, as well as the federal government, had health and safety legislation and regulations. The first was Saskatchewan under the guiding hand of a government administrator, Bob Sass, the Associate Deputy Minister of Health. He developed a framework for health and safety in Canada, much of which was adopted by the International Labour Organization (ILO) through a basic health and safety convention in 1981. Essentially, the framework consisted of three health and safety workers' rights: the right to participate, in the form of joint union-management health and safety committees, the right to refuse unhealthy and unsafe work and the right to know about workplace hazards. This was supplemented by a series of legally binding health and safety standards, limiting or eliminating workplace hazards.

From this framework, health and safety progressed further. There was a temptation to see health and safety solely in terms of workers' rights at the expense of standards: you could have a workplace rich in rights but still full of serious hazards. This meant that we had to balance rights with standards. Nor did health and safety committees have any real power without a strong union in the workplace, so we had to articulate and press for a relationship between health and safety bargaining and the work of joint committees. All this built upon Bob Sass' work.

At the same time, the focus of health and safety was changing. Union action had started as a campaign against physical injury and death but it became clear that there was a much bigger, hidden problem of occupational disease, largely unrecognized and uncompensated. So unions developed a program for addressing occupational diseases in addition to physical injuries, for which the causes and the action needed were much clearer. This focus on workplace diseases was later taken up anew when environmental protection was added to the occupational health and safety agenda.

FROM HEALTH AND SAFETY TO ENVIRONMENT

The Canadian Labour Congress (CLC) Environment Committee began as a sub-committee of the Occupational Health and Safety Committee in 1989. We produced a ten-point program for the environment, which called for workers' environmental rights, a worker perspective on the environment, stressed the connections between health and safety and environmental protection, and advocated a strong federal authority over the environment. We are still advocating.

Where did the pressure come from? There were two rank-and-file sentiments, which were rather distinct from each other. One comprised those who emphasized the connection between health and safety and the environment. The most obvious example was pollution: the pollutants that poison workers are also the toxins which erode community health outside the workplace and degrade the physical environment. The way that the CLC came to address the threefold issue of the health of the workplace, the community, and the environment was through an approach called Pollution Prevention. The aim of Pollution Prevention is to avoid the creation of pollutants in the first place, by preventing them from even entering the workplace as toxic chemical "inputs." In this way, "if it's not there, it can't pollute"—the workplace, the community, or the environment. This approach is contrasted with environmental control measures, in which there is an attempt to control the pollutants "at the end of the waste pipe," after they have been created and after they have contaminated the workplace.

The other grouping was more specifically environmental, in that it had an interest in the relationship between the workplace and the outside environment, rather than health and safety conditions within it. These union environmental activists saw environmental protection as a moral or political issue where workers had an interest, since workers were both polluters and the victims of pollution. The loyalties of such activists were equally to the union and the environment. I remember with great warmth, these early "labour environmentalists," such as Rick Coronado and Loretta Woodcock of the Canadian Auto Workers (CAW), Bob Diamond of the Newfoundland Association of Public Employees (NAPE), Helga Knote of the British Columbia Government Employees Union (BCGEU), Tom Wynn of the United Steelworkers (USW), and Mae Burrows of the United Fishers and Allied Workers Union (UFAWU) in British Columbia.

These labor environmental activists did their work at a time when few affiliated unions had environmental policies and no provision for the environment among union staff. They did not, on the whole, have to face the suspicion and skepticism that health and safety activists had to endure nearly a generation ago, but were regarded as somewhat odd, pursuing an issue which was not really of interest or concern to the union. However, the CAW, following the United Auto Workers (UAW) tradition, always did have a provision in its constitution that local unions must have an Environment Committee. Further, some unions, such as the International Woodworkers of America (IWA-Canada) did have policies on the sustainable environment that was necessary to maintain levels of employment. Nowadays, union policies on environment and energy are common, with environmental protection seen as a social value in its own right, not just a consequence of the need for jobs and work. There are also more functional policies on "green employment" or Green Job Creation. Again, most unions have a service provision for the environment, often as an extension of the Health and Safety Department. At the grass roots, the most effective labor organizations are the Regional Environmental Councils of the CAW.

The Environment Committee became a Standing Committee of the CLC at about the time I became Director in 1993. It was one of only six such CLC committees. Like other committees, it comprised union staff, a few union officers, and rank-and-file activists from public- and private-sector unions across the country. Considering the strength of the eco-feminist movement, it is surprising that there are and always have been relatively few women on the committee. The main issues to come before the committee concerned toxic chemicals and environmental pollution, reflecting the long-standing health and safety issue of workplace pollution. We did, however, get into the other two broad environmental issues which were natural resources and energy, both conservation and alternative energy sources. All these topics later coalesced in the new discipline and movement for sustainable development.

From the beginning, the committee worked in a way different from other CLC committees and, for that matter, most union committees in Canada. We created an Environmental Liaison Group, which comprised representatives from most of the national environmental groups and some regional ones. The members were invited to take part in Environment Committee meetings with voice but no vote (votes were rare in any case). Since the early 1990s, other union committees have followed suit, with social justice and other grass roots activists invited to committee meetings as "coalition partner."

The attempt to have the committee function as an arm of the environmental movement, as well as the labor movement was controversial. Some unionists objected to outsiders being privy to labor meetings. Others feared that the CLC's labor agenda would be submerged in the wider environmental movement and labor values nullified. There was one other major factor. The "war of the woods" was going on in British Columbia, particularly the bitter feud between Greenpeace and IWA-Canada. The committee and its driving force, CLC Executive Vice-President Dick Martin, were accused of siding with environmentalists against labor. Some demanded that the CLC stay out of forest issues completely. As a result, the CLC has avoided forest issues, apart from some important work on the Species at Risk Act. (There is, in any case, a minimal federal authority over forest policy.)

The committee demanded labor representation on every environmental issue, on every forum, so that labor was recognized as a constituency in its own right, with a distinct perspective. One result is that we took-on some issues that, in the scheme of things, weren't really very useful or significant. Another downside was that, to some in the labor movement, it seemed that we were more interested in butterflies, seals and spotted owls than in human beings and community health. Later, the committee developed much more of a human health slant on the issues, which increased our credibility within labour and which had a discernable impact on the approaches adopted by the wider environmental movement. The move also made it possible to see environmental protection as an integral part of social unionism.

How were we "labor environmentalists" regarded by the environmental movement? Some environmental leaders welcomed labor, particularly those in the bigger national environmental organizations. Others were suspicious, even hostile, regarding labor as allied to big polluters and colluding with the forest transnationals to attack environmentalists and screw the environment. Much of this sort of sentiment resided in the myriad of local environmental organizations, the core of the Canadian Environmental Network.

Our effectiveness consists largely in joining and working with such groups. Labor's part in pesticide action campaigns, cancer prevention coalitions and "toxics watch" groups has done much to overcome this suspicion and hostility. At the same time, and unlike social justice activists, relatively few environmentalists have been hired by the labor movement, activists such as Cliff Stainsby of the BCGEU and Diane Goulet of the Communication, Energy and Paperworkers' Union (CEP) being the exceptions.

The shift from ecological to human health issues was one positive move for labor. Another was the relationship between work and the environment. This should have been obvious from the start, but it was not. I plead that there was so much to learn about environmentalism that we could only develop a labor perspective when we understood all the dimensions of environmentalism itself.

The work-related environmental issues are twofold: Green Job Creation and Just Transition for Workers during Environmental Change. Logically, we should first have to create a host of green, clean, and healthy jobs, while concerning ourselves with workers who would lose their jobs in environmentally unsustainable industries. But this was not the way things worked in practice. The Just Transition movement (we can now call it that) started in the United States in the 1970s, the brainchild of the late Tony Mazzocchi of the Oil, Chemical and Atomic Workers (OCAW). Mazzocchi contended that American industry was so destructive to workers, the public and the environment that there was no alternative but to shut down huge segments of it altogether. Workers would be given compensation, education, and retraining to start a new life, much as veterans did after the Second World War. Since Mazzocchi's time, Just Transition has focused much more on industrial transformation rather than deindustrialization but his spirit lives on, the first and the greatest of all the labor environmentalists.

In Canada, Just Transition was taken up by the Energy and Chemical Workers Union (ECWU), then by the CEP (of which the ECWU was a founding component), then by the CLC. The common thread was in the person of Brian Kohler, who joined the CEP from the ECWU at the merger and made a major contribution to the CLC Just Transition policy, as did the Canadian Union of Public Employees (CUPE) and the United Steelworkers (USW). Just Transition has gained currency recently because of climate change and the alternative industries, particularly energy sources and energy efficiency, that are needed to implement the Kyoto Protocol. Here again, the CEP has been a leader, the first union to produce an energy policy and the union the most influential, with the CLC, of ensuring Canada's adoption of the Kyoto Protocol.

Just Transition has, however, remained largely a slogan and a well-articulated theoretical program. Why so? The reason is that industrial change in Canada has been slow and unimaginative. Had Canadian society and its government been in the vanguard of environmental change, we would by now (for instance) have had our own domestic wind power industry and wind power would be providing more of Canada's electricity. Workers who lost their jobs in redundant mines and ship repair facilities would be building wind towers and turbines—Just Transition in the best sense of the term. But this has not happened: Just Transition has not taken off because there has been no Green Job Creation worth the name.

For all that, environmentalism has enriched the labor movement. You cannot believe in a progressive industrial society without espousing an environmentalism which makes it truly progressive. Without the CLC, Pollution Prevention—this idea of preventing the creation of toxic pollutants instead of controlling them once created—would not have become the national environmental issue that it now is. To have been part of this movement, which is part labor, part environmental, and part "labor environmental" was, for me, the high point of 35 years in the labor movement.

PART II

Prevention versus Control: Early Moves

CHAPTER 3

Occupational Health: A Discipline Out of Focus

Here, I take occupational health to be a branch of environmental health in which the work environment assumes the place of the general environment in relation to the incidence of occupational disease. As such, "occupational health is, in many ways, just an environmental issue with an imaginary jurisdictional fence around it" [1]. But this fence is not merely arbitrarily placed; it has had consequences for the way in which scientific disciplines impinge on the practical discipline of improving and ensuring workers' health.

In this context, I take academic "science" in its usual dictionary definition so that it includes basic research in the search for truth. I also include, as science, those professional disciplines which depend on scientific truths for their success. Thus successful medicine depends, at least in part, on the truths of medical research and theoretical medicine. This is summed up in the term "scientific medicine." No doubt there are difficulties with such definitions, as there always will be when we try to define the relationship between objective truth and the related pragmatic disciplines in which objective truths are, in some way, applied. For instance, some professionals are students of both objective truth and practitioners of a pragmatic discipline such as occupational medicine. But, I submit, such problems are not great enough to subvert the arguments of this chapter which attempts to cast light on the proper relationship between scientific practitioners and a social issue such as occupational health [2].

We can illustrate the role of scientists in occupational health policy by examining three areas: the work of the International Commission on Radiological Protection (ICRP), the work in the area of chemical hazards of the American Conference of Governmental Industrial Hygienists Inc. (ACGIH), and the provisions of the International Labour Organization (ILO) Occupational Health Services Convention (1985). The first two of these cover worker exposure to ionizing radiations and to chemical substances respectively. All three cover a large area of occupational health (rather than safety) issues. Other health hazards

39

would include non-ionizing radiations, noise, vibration, stress, poor work design, and non-traumatic back injury (some of which are also dealt with by the ACGIH).

THE INTERNATIONAL COMMISSION ON RADIOLOGICAL PROTECTION (ICRP)

The ICRP issued its first report in 1928. The first quantitative radiation exposure limits were set in 1934. As a comment on the methodology of the ICRP and the availability of evidence, it is worth noting that the annual occupational exposure limit was reduced by a factor of nearly three from 1934 to 1950, by a further factor of three from 1950 to 1958, and by a further 60 percent from 1958 to 1991. In 1991, ICRP 60 reduced the whole body annual worker radiation "dose" limit from 50 milliSieverts (50mSv) to 20 mSv, though this figure could be averaged over a period of years. The 50 mSv limit lasted for a generation, from 1958 onwards, and survived the publication in 1977 of ICRP 26, which articulated a comprehensive radiation protection policy.

National governments broadly adopt the outlook and the recommendations of the ICRP, though with some variations, e.g., they may modify the recommendations regarding women workers on grounds of human rights or equity. The thinking of the ICRP has also found its way into the Codes of Practice of the ILO.

The term "Commission" suggests that some body, like a national government or an international agency, commissioned the ICRP to do work on its behalf and was answerable or accountable for its results. This term further suggests that the ICRP has executive as opposed to advisory powers. Neither of these is the case. Though national governments can, tacitly or explicitly, make recommendations as to the membership of the ICRP, it is, in fact, a self-appointed and self-perpetuating body of scientists, principally epidemiologists and health physicists. Epidemiology, using mainly atomic bomb data and e.g., health studies of uranium miners, is necessary to calculate the radiation risk estimates which form the bulk of the ICRP's work. But health physics is also needed because the ICRP uses biological reasoning in calculating the health effects of different types of radiation and translating them into a single "effective dose."

Radiation protection is based on two principles:

1. The calculation of numerical exposure limits; and
2. The ALARA principle that doses should be As Low As Reasonably Achievable, economic and social factors being taken into account.

The ICRP acknowledges that both of these entail value judgments as well as the use of scientific concepts. In setting a numerical limit, the ICRP makes comparisons with other (hazardous) occupations and makes moral inferences about the acceptability of risk compared with the degree of risk in other occupations. Similarly, ALARA means making judgments as to the importance in policy-making of economic and social values.

Behind both principles lies a scientific theory as to the general relationship between exposure and effects on health (principally cancer and reproductive damage). The first part of the theory says that the relationship between dose and detriment is linear-quadratic, i.e., there is a direct and uniform relationship between the amount of radiation to which workers are exposed and the detriments to the health of those workers as a group (technically, a "population"). One consequence is that, for instance, a given number of units of dosage spread around a given number of workers will have the same health effects as half the given dose spread around double the number of workers. If the units of dosage remain the same, the detriments (e.g., the number of cancers) will remain the same, whether they are "spread around" a higher or a lower number of workers. Thus it is no use reducing individual dosage if the "collective dose" remains the same. Any one individual's risk is reduced, but at the price of increasing (directly) the number of workers at risk. The only really effective way of reducing risk is to reduce the number of units of actual exposure.

The second part of the theory says that there is no threshold or lower limit below which radiation exposure is safe. All radiation exposure, in other words, is bad. A reduction in exposure from 50 to 45 units will have the same health effects as a reduction in exposure from 6 units to 1 unit: there is no point at the lower end of the scale where a reduction in exposure will lead to a dramatic improvement in workers' health [3].

Both these principles are based on inferences from actual exposure data, e.g., there will be much more evidence based on exposures around 50 mSv than there is from exposures around 5 mSv. But the inferences are so widely and strongly held that the two principles are accepted as axioms guiding radiation policy. Contentions, for instance, that since the human race has survived quite happily with small doses of "background" radiation, a "little radiation may be good for you," are usually put forward flippantly and polemically. No one seriously proposes that radiation workers ought to be exposed to a little radiation as a positive matter of public policy, since almost everyone holds that a little radiation is a little bad, and there is no safe lower limit.

Faced with these principles, lay critics of the ICRP's work have basically three choices. First, they could enter the scientific debate, for instance, by publishing articles on the risk estimates which are subject to peer review. This is difficult but not impossible to do. For instance, ICRP methodology could be criticized by saying that the Commission should consider all epidemiological studies, not just the central ones, however shoddy or inconclusive such studies may be. This "meta-epidemiology" would use sophisticated statistical techniques and would likely result in a higher estimate of radiation risk [4]. But unless such a scientific insight were delivered in the context of a thorough knowledge of the literature (to a Ph.D. level of competence), it would not likely find its way into the radiation literature. Even more important, the number of articles making points of this kind would be dwarfed by publications of the conventional kind at a time when the number of citations in the literature is being used as a criterion of interest and competence [5].

Second, they could criticize not the quality of the science but the scientific strategy adopted by the ICRP. For instance, the ALARA principle is advanced merely as a definition or as a slogan; it is not spelled out as a practical way of minimizing radiation exposure. It would be quite possible to produce a number of "practical paradigms," detailing the best industrial practice, e.g., in the design and operation of X-ray equipment, nuclear plant maintenance, plant component shielding, the manufacture of radioisotopes, the handling of "hot" nuclear components, etc., and offering these as *by definition* reasonably achievable. Despite disclaimers in the Annals of the ICRP, the chief device for radiation protection is still in the form of dose limits rather than in the much lower levels of exposure that could be achieved by giving substance to ALARA. After all, if all radiation is dangerous, the practical minimization of dose is much more important than the analysis of evidence and the determination of outer dose limits which is derived from it. If, for example, there is *no* point at which the nuclear industry is declared to be too dangerous for people to work in it, it is worth asking whether the numerical limits should form part of a viable strategy at all since an ALARA principle with substance will always be more protective than a numerical limit [6].

Lastly, the public could dismiss the work of the ICRP as ideology. This is not the same as suggesting that "science is for sale" [7], which is the contention that employers bend or otherwise influence the results of scientific inquiry, e.g., by testing the workplace for the wrong contaminants and then declaring it "clean!" The contention that science is ideology is different and stronger. Essentially, this view says that the social perspective of scientific researchers determines the conclusions of the scientific enterprise.

In the case of the ICRP, the argument would state that the Commissioners are members of a professional middle class who depend, for their social status and their role in society, on the existence of the multi-trillion dollar nuclear fuel cycle. Their scientific activity will ensure that they are entrenched in the radiation protection business in such a way that they will never work themselves out of a job nor produce conclusions which can be handed over to the public and made the property of the interested parties. In short, the ICRP exercises hegemony over radiation protection: an unelected and unaccountable body sets the social agenda without the force of law or the law of force.

While this argument may succeed as a sociological analysis, it does not prove the point that its proponents want to make: namely, that there is no such thing as objective scientific fact, only expressions of the hegemony of one social group or class (or its members). It may be quite true that if another social group (such as workers) exercised hegemony, there would be better research, more of it, or that it would be more influential in setting progressive social policy. But proponents of the argument want to say more than this: they want to say that *all* science is ideological and that none of it has a characteristic called objectivity whereby something is true independently of which social group adheres to it. Thus declarations like "when we get into power, we will get the sort of science we deserve and which prove the points we want to make" are capable of two interpretations. The first, that science will get better, is not controversial even if it is not true. The second interpretation is that all science is ideological which would leave one wondering why its practitioners would bother to engage in it at all since its results would be (according to the theory) a foregone conclusion. In the case of the nuclear fuel cycle, they would forget the charade of research which is merely a sociological phenomenon and either minimize the hazards to nuclear operators or simply close the whole industry down [8]. The argument of this chapter, by contrast, is not that there is no such thing as objective science, but rather, there is a question of how, if at all, such science is used in implementing social policy and of who should make such decisions—by implication, not scientists themselves.

THE AMERICAN CONFERENCE OF GOVERNMENTAL INDUSTRIAL HYGIENISTS (ACGIH)

One of the central functions of the ACGIH is to produce a list (revised annually) of numerical Threshold Limit Values (TLVs) which "represent conditions under which it is believed that nearly all workers may be reasonably exposed day after day without adverse effect" [9]. In other words, the table of numbers (exposure limits) for several hundred airborne substances are believed to be safe for the vast majority of workers exposed to them. The texts of ACGIH make it clear that industrial diseases contracted by the remainder are due essentially to some cause other than the permitted exposure [10].

Like the ICRP, the ACGIH is well established, having been founded in 1938. Despite the title, the "Conference is a professional society, not an official Government Agency." Nor is membership restricted to hygienists; it is open to professional personnel in government agencies and educational institutions engaged in occupational safety and health programs. There are more than 3,000 members from the United States and around the world. The organization is neither peculiarly American, particularly limited to hygiene, nor governmental.

The Chemical Substances TLV Committee, for instance, is comprised of members with qualifications in medicine, industrial hygiene, engineering, and science. Some are academics, others are employed in the public sector, e.g., by the armed forces and municipalities. The medical representation is particularly strong among the Consultants to the Committee, many of whose members are employed by private corporations.

Recently, there have been two sorts of criticism of the ACGIH TLVs. One of these says that, scientifically, the TLVs are not really thresholds at all, a claim made among others by S. A. Roach, D.Sc., Ph.D., and S. M. Rappaport, Ph.D. [11]. The other claims a corporate influence on the construction of TLVs, e.g., the Consultants to the TLV Committee were given primary responsibility for developing TLVs on proprietary chemicals of the companies that employed them. The epitome of such influence is through the work of company doctors. This claim is made by B. I. Castleman, Sc.D., and G. E. Ziem, M.D. [12].

It is important to understand exactly what is being said by the critics of TLVs, particularly on the question of how far TLVs serve corporate interests. Roach and Rappaport, for instance, point out that TLVs are constructed on the basis of actual industrial practice (i.e., of existing levels of contamination), thus legitimizing the *status quo*. This means, in practice, that TLVs are not purely "health-based" (as claimed), but represent a compromise between health and industrial practice. Castleman and Ziem point out the extreme scarcity, unevenness, and low quality of the scientific evidence on which TLVs are supposed to be based. Above all, they showed that, in a number of cases, the limits were set by staff of the companies producing the chemicals on, at best, anecdotal evidence with no dissent from the TLV Committee.

None of these critics suggest that employers have deliberately perverted scientific inquiry or scientific results, the accusation that "science is for sale."

This being so, there seem to be two distinct complaints about TLVs which can be examined quite separately: the contention that TLVs represent poor science and the contention that they are subject to corporate influence. The latter contention necessarily implies the former (otherwise the corporate influence would be without substance); but the former could well be true without the latter. There is also a third possibility (a version, in a way, of corporate influence): that employers and others have accepted, uncritically, modes of scientific advice which entrench workplace pollution and which do not result in the most effective strategies for promoting occupational health [13].

There are, in fact, three sorts of strategy which could be adopted by the public in response to complaints about TLVs and the ways in which they are set. The first is to insist that evidence is collected by some body which is independent of any interest, corporate or otherwise. For instance, workers have been held to have a right to independent medical advice from sources not beholden in any way to employers, i.e., from sources other than company doctors.

On paper, this is the position taken by many critics of TLVs; but, in practice, they want standards to be set by another group of scientists, e.g., the progressive scientists who comprise some of the membership of the international Collegium Ramazzini. This body is certainly independent of employers, but commentators may observe that it is a voluntary scientific body like ICRP and ACGIH with no more mandate to make policy recommendations than any other.

The second is to insist on a proper scientific procedure for setting exposure limits by detailing the range of evidence as a necessary basis for positing a limit, by stipulating the procedures (e.g., air monitoring) to be used in collecting such information, and the range of health effects which will be considered in trying to discern a detriment.

This procedure is controversial. For instance, it is practically impossible to insist on the huge range of evidence of the sort which is presently available for asbestos. The practical range of evidence would be much more restricted, e.g., to toxicity data. It would also have to be uniform for each chemical; otherwise, the limits chosen would be based on inconsistent ranges of evidence, one of Castleman and Ziem's well-founded complaints. So agreement would have to be reached on what sort of evidence has to be generated and considered, principally toxicity tests. This agreement would constitute a value judgment and there is no special reason why scientists should be a party to such policy decision-making.

Then there would have to be agreement on criteria for relating both evidence and detriments to policy [14]. By this, I mean that the different sorts of evidence, e.g., the different sorts of toxicity tests, and their results, would have to be weighted in regard to each other as well as in relation to the limit set (the "regulatory outcome"). Technically, this can be described as a mapping exercise in which the values determined for each sort of test (each sort of evidence), such as Lethal Dose test result or a positive/negative (yes/no) result in a mutagenicity test, are "mapped onto" a scale of outcomes, i.e., the ranges for exposure limits. Such criteria are entirely absent from TLV methodology. Again, they constitute a non-scientific value judgment.

The criteria have to meet scientific considerations of aptitude, e.g., it is no use basing a limit largely on the inhalation route of exposure when the main route of "uptake" is through skin absorption. And they have to meet logical requirements of consistency: the same mapping scheme has to apply equally to all chemicals. But, this being said, the question of "how much protection are workers to get in the light of the evaluation scheme?" is a question of values, not of scientific fact. "How the scheme is applied to the practical reality of the workplace" is not a scientific matter, simply because the scheme can be applied in non-arbitrary ways to offer more or to offer less protection, according to political decision.

Faced with the practical and socioeconomic complexities of such a program, critics may opt for a third choice, namely to set limits on a pragmatic basis looking to best industrial practice and the most stringent limits adopted in practice by industrialized countries and particular industries—on the assumption that all exposures are likely to be harmful, and the smaller they are, the better. Scientific reasoning could still be used in determining the priorities for minimizing exposures to various chemicals but without any need to know whether the priorities are grounded in scientific certainties. All we have to have is agreement that such-and-such a class of evidence will be used to determine such-and-such a priority for instituting prevention measures, which is a rational procedure but not, in itself, a scientific one. For instance, we may have to decide whether a potential carcinogen is of more concern than an actual mutagen (again suitably defined). But, whatever we do, there will be political choices and political, not scientific, decisions to be made [15].

The strategy of pursuing "pragmatic limits" is to be contrasted with the strategy of "practising industrial hygiene with no limits." The latter rests on the premise that TLVs are so deeply flawed that the whole approach to industrial health, based on numerical exposure limits, has to be abandoned in favor of a valid and more efficacious approach.

In some ways, such proposals are less radical than they first appear. Eileen Senn Tarlau [16], for instance, has proposed a scheme of "no limits," but, in the course of explicating it, she makes it clear that she supports a new set of limits which are now called Health-Based Exposure Limits (HBELs). A number of researchers, including Ziem and Castleman, took a large amount of data used by the Environmental Protection Agency, together with standard risk assessment methods, to yield a new set of limits much tighter (lower) than TLVs [17].

This procedure still embodies (non-scientific) values and it still raises issues about the propriety of scientists laying claim to the best approach to workers' health. The procedure is also based on the traditional premise that some exposures are legitimate until scientific evidence compels us to alter the exposure limits (almost always downwards).

The procedure is radical in two main ways. First, the numerical values are based on the idea that workers are entitled to the same standards of protection as the general public and the physical environment. Second, compared with common industrial practice, some of the limits amount virtually to Zero Exposure [18] in the workplace [19]. In this respect, the strategy shifts away from numerical limits to the practical minimization of exposures wherever feasible.

There is a clear strain to this effect in the writings of both E. S. Tarlau and Ziem and Castleman. Tarlau, for instance, refers to the need for "checking on control measures" and on observing work processes as they are actually carried out. Ziem and Castleman emphasize that:

> . . . air monitoring should be used to assess the effectiveness of controls. In addition, because at this time there are no known safe exposure levels, physicians as part of the management team should insist on controls that reduce all exposures to the *maximum extent technically feasible.* To advocate a lesser degree of protection would violate the dictum to "do no harm." [20]

If this is done, we can see a definite and welcome shift in the traditional approach to occupational health. But if we are really to make progress toward reducing exposures to "the maximum extent technically feasible," there will have to be a yardstick by which progress can actually be measured. It is hard to see how this can be done without, at least, some interim pragmatic exposure limits of the sort described earlier.

There is a second query. The emphasis on control measures suggests that the technical expertise needed is essentially engineering in character, leaving very little room for the medical profession and the associated industrial hygiene. Yet, Tarlau and Ziem and Castleman continue to envisage a strong role for the medical profession in workplaces, the latter suggesting that "workers have been ill-served by having critical decisions about their health delegated to engineers carrying TLV booklets" [21]. To the role of physicians in occupational health, we must now turn.

THE ILO OCCUPATIONAL HEALTH SERVICES CONVENTION

The ILO Convention concerning Occupational Health Services (1985) [22] is important because it raises issues concerning the *prevention* of industrial diseases as opposed to monitoring them or dealing with them once workers have contracted them.

In environmental protection, which is the protection of the physical environment (and sometimes also the human communities outside the workplace), the distinction between prevention and the *control* of environmental hazards is, by now, well established [23]. The prevention of pollution means the prevention of the production of environmental pollutants so that they cannot damage the environment. This can be achieved by banning the production of certain pollutants or by changing industrial processes so that they are not produced during a manufacturing or other type of production. The control of pollutants, on the other hand, means the management or mitigation of pollution once it has been produced, e.g., by installing control measures "at the end of the pipe." Prevention, according to environmental science, is more effective than control [24].

In occupational health, the distinction between prevention and control has been, traditionally, far less clear—one pernicious consequence of the "imaginary jurisdictionary fence" built around workplace health and safety. The control of hazards "at the source" has been advocated by professional practitioners, and it is invariably conceded that control at the source of the hazard, e.g., by the Total Enclosure or Total Isolation of an industrial process, is the most effective control method [25]. However, the banning of specified chemical substances has also been advocated and practiced, which would count as a prevention measure in environmental thinking. Workplace control measures do not necessarily protect the outside environment, since workers can be insulated from dangerous chemicals which, nevertheless, pollute the environment beyond the "end of the pipe."

In occupational health, a less controversial distinction is between prevention/control measures on one side (to the extent that control fulfills the aims of prevention in regard to workplace pollution), and *remedial* measures which deal with industrial diseases once they have been contracted. The surveillance of workers' health, workers' compensation, counseling (e.g., over hearing loss), first aid, occupational nursing services, and medical services all count (with some reservations, to be discussed below) as remedial action rather than prevention/control.

I am going to take it as axiomatic that preventive action is always preferable to remedial action in protecting workers' health. Sometimes, preventive action is more costly in the short run than remedial measures, and the whole question of cost (as opposed to net health benefit) is distorted because it is easier for employers to "externalize" the costs of ill health (i.e., to have someone else pay for them) than it is to find someone else to foot the bill for truly preventive measures.

There is a further distinction which has to be understood in order to get ILO "instruments" into perspective. "Performance standards" are those which specify an outcome (a standard to be met) but which do not specify the means, e.g., within a workplace, by which the outcome is to be met. "Specification standards," on the other hand, specify the means by which an outcome is to be achieved, such as the institution of a specified process within an industrial plant. Sometimes a specification standard is implied rather than stated. For instance, a regulation requiring the Zero Discharge of dioxins from a pulp mill can be complied with only by banning chlorine and chlorinated compounds from the production process. Instead of banning chlorine and chlorinated compounds from mills (a specification standard), a performance standard is instituted which implies a specification.

This distinction is helpful as far as it goes; but it does not tell the whole story, since there is an equally important distinction between types of outcome or performance. For instance, in health and safety, a standard embodied in regulation might require "adequate toilets" in a workplace. On the other hand, a standard might require, instead, X number of toilets per Y number of employees on duty at any one time. The latter is clearer and much easier to enforce.

Another example: a law may require chemical supplier companies to disclose the chemical names of the ingredients of their products to an extent which is adequate to identify the principle hazards of the products subject to business confidentiality. Alternatively, the law could require the disclosure of the chemical names of all the ingredients unless the ingredients are subject individually to an explicit claim of trade secrecy, to be adjudicated by the regulatory authority.

In both these examples, the former case could be labeled a performance standard and the latter a specification standard. If this is done, we still have to be clear that the problem is with the vagueness of the outcome. Numerical exposure limits are precise performance standards while industrial process standards are specification standards but without necessarily any specified outcome.

In general, ILO *Conventions* contain performance standards and imprecise outcomes while ILO *Recommendations* contain more specification standards. For instance, the ILO Convention on Safety in the Use of Asbestos contains less firm rules about the banning and restriction of certain forms of asbestos than the parallel Recommendation.

These distinctions are essential if we are to understand the thrust of the ILO Convention on Occupational Health Services.

The Conventions and Recommendations of the ILO are produced through tripartite discussions between representatives of employers, workers, and national governments, then adopted by the governing bodies of the ILO which comprise, again, representatives of the three constituencies. The ILO is unique in the UN in recognizing the authority (as opposed to the advice) of parties other than governments. Governments, clearly, are responsible for health matters within their borders, including occupational health. Workers have a special interest (and perhaps, as such, an exclusive interest) in conditions of work, which includes health and safety.

The role of employers is less clear since, in a sense, they create the problems of health and safety. I say "in a sense" because there will always be problems of health and safety in industrial enterprises to some extent, irrespective of who the employer is, i.e., whether the employer is private, public, or the workers collectively (a cooperative).

But once we acknowledge that health and safety is a socioeconomic matter involving decisions about the economic utility of regulatory and other action, we have to acknowledge that employers have an interest in this area. Where there are value judgments there will be a legitimate clash of values which the organs of the ILO aim to reconcile.

Conventions of the ILO are adopted voluntarily by national governments; this is the next stage after adoption by the ILO governing bodies. Recommendations remain as Recommendations.

Most Conventions trail behind the common industrial practice of (most) First World countries and, since they usually comprise performance standards., they do not impose heavy obligations either on governments or on business (or on workers, for that matter). But it is difficult to fault the process by which they are framed. In cases where UN agencies produce more stringent standards (embedded, e.g., in the work of the World Health Organization), they do not have the authority or the public focus of the ILO governing bodies.

The ILO Convention on Occupational Health Services requires governments to have a policy on occupational health services. The text of the Convention makes it clear that such services are to be *within* workplaces. Personnel of health services are to be employees of an employer and only coincidentally, in some cases, employees of governments. The Convention has provisions to protect the "professional independence" of health service personnel (Article 10), and there are provisions protecting the confidentiality of medical information on employees (Recommendations 11-18).

The Convention makes many stipulations about the work of occupational health services, including workplace surveillance and the planning, organization, and design of work (Article 5). However, a central function is the surveillance of workers' health in relation to work (Article 5[f]; Recommendations 11-12).

Reflecting these facts, it is understandable that occupational health services should be multidisciplinary (Article 9[1]; Recommendation 36). However, when we look at the work to be undertaken by occupational health services, we see that it includes risk identification and assessment (Article 5[a]). This is clearly a technical research matter, and indeed research, e.g., for epidemiological purposes, is clearly advocated (Recommendation 30). When this is combined with the worker health surveillance provisions, we can see that despite the ideal of prevention (Recommendation 3), the composition of occupational health services is weighted toward the *remedial* as opposed to the prevention/control side of health and safety.

This is verified when we look at the examples given of the multidisciplinary team: occupational medicine, occupational hygiene, ergonomics, and occupational health nursing (Recommendation 36[2]). Of these, only ergonomics is clearly a preventive discipline. There is also a stress on the need for appropriate scientific and technical knowledge in order to perform the duties relevant to these fields (Recommendation 36[2]).

With this slant toward the remedial side of occupational health, it is worth asking what the proper role of medicine and related disciplines ought to be.

Doctors treat people for injury, disease, and general malaise. The current emphasis on preventive medicine only points to this fact, and to the gross imbalance between resources devoted to prevention as opposed to remedial treatment.

At the same time, it is clear that the medical profession has established itself in a pivotal position in regard to workplace health, e.g., on the TLV Committee, where MDs far outnumber professional engineers. The senior health and safety official in a workplace is often a medical doctor, even though the training available in occupational medicine may be minimal.

Things were not always this way. Before concern about workplace disease superseded concern about traumatic injury, the relevant professionals were industrial engineers, e.g., in the work of the Canadian Standards Association. Societies of safety engineers survive. The main focus of such engineering activity was, however, on such things as machinery guarding, electrical safety, and personal protective equipment, not on industrial design and ergonomics. Engineers had also the reputation of being politically conservative.

When industrial disease became the prime concern [26], there seems to have been a natural association of disease with the work of physicians who, as a body, had the reputation of being politically progressive (medicine is a Good Thing after all).

Though physicians are concerned primarily with treatment, there is an ideology of occupational disease prevention which is sometimes used to legitimize the role of physicians in the occupational health disciplines. This takes the form of the doctrine of Primary, Secondary, and Tertiary Prevention [27]. Primary Prevention is prevention "at the source" of the industrial hazard and the denial of work to those liable to suffer particularly from industrial health hazards. Secondary Prevention is the early diagnosis of a disease and the arrest of its subsequent progress. Tertiary Prevention consists in making a patient comfortable once a disease has taken hold.

This doctrine is curious, to say the least. "Medical removal" from work occurs in order to reduce the risk of disease arising from a particular work hazard. Almost always, medical removal takes the form not of reducing hazard exposure overall but by rotating work among a pool of workers. For instance, when a worker in a lead smelter gets "leaded," s/he is removed and another gets put in her/his place. In such cases, one worker's removal is another worker's poison. We could, indeed, see a potential reduction in the incidence of industrial disease if there were some "threshold of risk" or a low point in the dose-response curve to which the pool of workers gravitated in contrast with exposure at the dangerous, high points on the curve. But, as we have seen, such contentions are a very weak point in the science of industrial hygiene.

Specifically, the dose-response curve for ionizing radiation is a straight line while thresholds are generally speculative at best. Medical removal is thus a preventive measure only in a Pickwickian sense: anyone can prevent industrial disease if there is no industry or industry idle for want of workers.

Secondary and Tertiary Prevention are really only Treatment under another name, leaving us with prevention/control at the source as the only genuine part of the ideology.

And when we look at the sort of prevention measures needed to give substance to Primary Prevention, we find that doctors have neither the technical qualifications (in engineering) nor the authority in the workplace to carry them out. We can only conclude that employers genuinely interested in prevention have succumbed so deeply to medical expertise that they devote resources toward the least effective strategies for promoting occupational health.

These resources are considerable since an occupational health service worth the name can cost a medium-sized employer several hundred thousand dollars a year and more. One can buy a lot of preventive engineering for a million dollars a year.

DISCUSSION AND CONCLUSION

In all three of the areas discussed, there are serious flaws in the approach to the health issues concerned. With radiation protection, there are some possible criticisms of the science which is practiced but, moreover, there are deep faults in the scientific strategy for protecting workers' health. A strategy based on taking the ALARA principle seriously would result in far more effective protection than first positing a principle of "acceptable risk," then positing some science-based numerical exposure limits supposedly compatible with the acceptable risk articulated or assumed.

With the ACGIH TLVs there are, in contrast, some deep criticisms of the scientific procedure which is utilized to yield the numerical values; but some of these flaws are shared by all procedures which try to relate bodies of evidence to prescriptive conclusions about permitted exposures. Hence, it is better to look at exposure limits as pragmatic rather than science-based if, indeed, it is worth adopting the notion of permissible numerical limits at all.

Both the ICRP and the ACGIH adopt the notion of an acceptable limit to workplace health rather than a *minimization strategy* which aims to reduce workplace hazards to the lowest feasible level.

The criticism of the ILO instruments is rather different. As with the ICRP and ACGIH, scientific and moral values are embedded in the texts of the instruments, but the medical profession can hardly be faulted if the stakeholders (the three parties to the ILO) choose to encapsulate these values in their deliberations. The fact that a second-best strategy (remediation rather than prevention) has been adopted is not because the ILO has accorded any special place to medical and scientific interests.

This point could be generalized. It is governments, employers, and workers who make policy. If they choose to adopt misguided strategies emanating from the scientific and medical community, so much the worse for them.

Nevertheless, the point remains: the scientific and moral values of scientists have a strong influence on occupational health policy, giving a misdirected thrust to the practice of the discipline. In other words, it is scientists who are responsible for a discipline out of focus. We should ask why this is so and what the future of scientific hegemony is likely to be.

We live in a "scientific culture." This means that policy-makers such as governments, employers, and (collectively) workers look to science as a basis of policy or as a justification for the policies which are adopted. Physicians, toxicologists, hygienists, epidemiologists, risk analysts, and health physicists are, in this sense, all "scientists" according to the loose definition adopted at the beginning of this chapter.

There ought to be a clear distinction between the facts or the objective truths of science on one hand and, on the other, the prescriptions, policies, and strategies which are, in some way, related to them [28].

But, I contend, this is not so, since *de facto*, the science which is appealed to, embodies both moral values and the strategies which will be used in the approach to industrial disease. These prescriptive issues ought to be for (democratic) policy-makers to decide. If I am correct, the strategies have, in effect, already been decided before the policy process takes place—to the detriment of truly effective policies to promote and protect workers' health.

Even when the professionals "get it right"—and some of the sources discussed in this piece clearly do—there is still a further question as to the status of the source of the advice. Is the source to be respected as a professional or simply as the voice of one educated citizen among many? In other words, which constituency does the voice represent? (The idea that the voice is the voice of "science" is of no help in deciding the proper foundations of policy.)

There is the beginning of a social tendency to recognize a "scientific constituency" as such. For instance, the United Nations recognizes a number of interests, "major groups" or "social partners," in addition to national governments. These include women, youth, Indigenous Peoples, non-government organizations (NGOs), trade unions, local authorities—and "the scientific and technological community" [29]. Apart from workers and employers in the ILO, these groups have, however, only advisory powers. In Canada, academics and scientists are given a distinct place in public consultations over environmental and health policy. It is hard to see what interests such individuals represent. If they do not (and perhaps cannot) represent the discipline called "science," they must represent the interests and powers of scientists in society which, I have suggested, stand in need of vindication.

I want to conclude by making some remarks about the nature of occupational health as a discipline. If we endorse the distinction between the preventive and the remedial sides of industrial health and accord primacy to the former, there will indeed be a firm place for the health-related disciplines [30]; but there will be an even more central place for industrial engineers. Engineers enjoy a bad reputation in occupational health and, as has been seen, some of this reputation is deserved. This is unfortunate because engineering suitably construed, and not medicine, is the key to occupational health.

This being so, I suggest that the proper profile of a contemporary occupational health technician would involve expertise in:

1. those techniques which industrial process engineers traditionally need to produce high-quality products efficiently;
2. engineering techniques aimed at the prevention of occupational disease;
3. the techniques of safety engineering, but focused on the design of work processes rather than, e.g., personal protective equipment; and
4. techniques which are aimed at the prevention of environmental hazards, e.g., pollution prevention rather than control.

The first of these techniques involves two sorts of expertise. One consists of answers to the question "Does the process do what it is supposed to do?" This is a question of industrial effectiveness, e.g., in producing high-quality products. The second consists of answers to the question "Does the process do well, what it is supposed to do?" This is a question of industrial efficiency, e.g., production with minimum energy consumption and minimum waste. Industries can be effective but inefficient and vice-versa. There may also be a third question "Can the engineer decide on which products to produce?" This is a less traditional question but one which is pertinent, simply because some engineers do decide on products. The model of success in the computer hardware industry is the engineer-entrepreneur. There may also be other prominent cases, e.g., in the motor industry, where engineer-managers such as Lee Iacocca decide on "which products to produce." This is in an industry where there is no clear distinction between an object and its design. For instance, a "compact car" must be designed in specific ways or it will not count as a compact car.

The first and fourth of these techniques are starting to be combined, i.e., in such a way that industrial efficiency and environmental protection are to be regarded wherever possible as two faces of the same coin. Where this is not being done, it is reckoned to take two years to train a chemical engineer so as to meet the joint requirements of these two poles. This leaves us with two major disciplines which, up to now, have been independent, namely safety engineering and what passes for occupational disease prevention. Training technicians in a new four-fold discipline is, therefore, a tall order. But it is essential if we are to make a genuine inroad into the problem of industrial disease. As it is, the discipline of occupational health is out of focus, partly because the strategies which inform it are misguided and partly because remediation is emphasized to the virtual exclusion of disease prevention.

REFERENCES

1. See Schrecker, T. *CLC/NRTEE Handbook on Sustainable Development,* where Brian Kohler of the Energy and Chemical Workers Union is quoted on p. 38 of the draft.
2. There is almost no discussion in this chapter of the relationship between objective truths or facts and prescriptive values, an ethical or philosophical issue. Nor is there any discussion of the relationship between the different sorts and aims of science and its practitioners, i.e., scientists.
3. The two parts of the theory of ionizing radiation are summarized in "Radiation and Radioactive Materials" by Hobbs, Charles H., and McClellan, Roger O., in *Toxicology, The Basic Study of Poisons,* 2nd edition, edited by John Doull, M.D., Ph.D., C. D. Klassen, Ph.D., and M. O. Amdur, Ph.D., Macmillan, 1980, pp. 515-516.
4. For a step in this direction, see *Submission of the Canadian Labour Congress to the Atomic Energy Control Board on Proposed Revisions to Regulations* under the Atomic Energy Control Act, January 1984.
5. National scientific competence is being measured by the number of citations in the scientific literature. It would be easy to do a similar exercise detailing the academic qualifications and the occupations of the contributors.
6. Unions have given substance to ALARA through collective bargaining—not by reference to ALARA in the law but by negotiating limits which are significantly lower than the ICRP doses. Unions which have attempted this, with varying degrees of success, include the United Steelworkers of America, the Canadian Union of Public Employees (especially the Ontario Hydro Employees' Union, CUPE Local 1000) and the Oil, Chemical and Atomic Workers International Union.
7. See e.g. Sass, B. *The Work Environment Board and the Limits of Democracy,* note 37; forthcoming.
8. This argument cannot be annotated since it is so rarely articulated or, in the contemporary literature, written down. At least one origin of the argument is to be found in the Stalinist literature of about 1945 onwards, particularly on genetics and philology. It is also difficult to reconstruct because, I believe, it is incoherent.
9. See the booklet, published annually, *Threshold Limit Values and Biological Exposure Indices.*
10. See the Introduction to the booklet cited in note 9 above.

11. Roach, S. A., and Rappaport, S. M . But They Are Not Thresholds: A Critical Analysis of the Documentation of Threshold Limit Values, *American Journal of Industrial Medicine, 17*, pp. 717-753, 1990.

12. Castleman, B. I., and Ziem, G. E. Corporate Influence on TLVs, *American Journal of Industrial Medicine, 13,* pp. 531-559, 1998.

13. This is not the place to examine the role of science in business ideology. But one common business ploy (it is not the only one) is to insist on "good science" in the formulation of environmental policy. As such, this is a conflation of two ideas: (1) that we should utilize science, and science of good quality; and (2) that such science should serve the public good. Both of these themes are examined below. I make a distinction between the pursuit of good science, which is not controversial, and the choice of *scientific strategies* which, for practical purposes like occupational health, is not in itself a scientific matter in that science itself cannot tell us which strategies to adopt. In practice, businesses often advocate scientific strategies which are inconclusive or which legitimize the status quo (pretty much the same thing). They can then claim that policy rests on good science which in sense (1) above, it may well do. The reader must decide whether environmental health policy is driven more by business ideology (often called corporate interests) or more generally by the implied choice of scientific strategies. This chapter points to the latter rather than the former.

14. Such a scheme for chemical pesticides is sketched out in Bennett, D. "Pesticide Reduction, A Case Study from Canada," *New Solutions,* Fall 1991, pp. 59-63.

15. In considering all of the alternative strategies, it is possible to overestimate the divergences from TLVs. For instance, while TLVs may come from private industry in the ways detailed by the critics, they are adopted, sometimes with variations, by many national and sub-national governments as a matter of public policy. Other countries have different sorts of limits such as Maximum Acceptable Concentrations (MACs) or Permitted Exposure Limits (PELs). But they are set in ways comparable to TLVs and there is not always a high degree of divergence from the numerical TLV values. Even when countries have a process for modifying PELs after the scientists have put forward their recommendations (as happens, e.g., in the Netherlands and the Nordic countries), the rationale for setting limits remains similar to that of TLVs, with scientists determining the approach and setting the basis of the public agenda. The argument of this chapter suggests that the search for genuine thresholds in an agreed scientific sense is clumsy, time-consuming, and expensive, with no guarantee of success. Meanwhile, workers continue to be poisoned *en masse.*

16. See Tarlau, Eileen Senn, "Industrial Hygiene with No Limits," *American Industrial Hygiene Association Journal, 51,* pp. A-9 to A-10, January 1990.

17. Tarlau, op. cit., p. A-9; Ziem, M.D., Grace E., and Castleman, Sc.D., Barry I., "Threshold Limit Values: Historical Perspectives and Current Practice," *Journal of Occupational Medicine, 31*:11, November 1989; the Health-Based Exposure Limits Committee, *Health-Based Exposure Limits,* Draft 6, October 28, 1991.

18. Zero Exposure to workplace carcinogens has been the official policy of the Canadian Labour Congress since 1984 and, in one guise or another, even further back than that.

19. The 1991 values for HBELs are, in many cases, far lower than the "three or more orders of magnitude" cited by Ziem and Castleman, op. cit., three years earlier.

20. Tarlau, op. cit., p. A-10; Ziem and Castleman, op. cit., p. 916.

21. Ziem and Castleman, op. cit., p. 917. The authors point to the need to monitor exposures and the health of workers and for industrial physicians to have the authority to fulfill their professional obligations to the people at work. They also couple two ideas: (1) respect on the part of employers for the importance of industrial medicine, with (2) managerial commitment to prevent industrial diseases. In regard to industrial hygienists, Tarlau emphasizes that professionals must routinely talk to workers as "the best source of what is happening in the workplace;" they must also conduct interviews of workers in order to understand and evaluate the state of the workers' health (Tarlau, op. cit., p. A-10).

22. Convention No. 161: Convention concerning Occupational Health Services (1985) coming into force 17 February 1988. Recommendation No. 171: Recommendation concerning Occupational Health Services.

23. See e.g., Commoner, Barry. *Making Peace With the Planet,* Pantheon Books, New York, 1990, Chapter 3; Rossi, Mark, Ellenbecker, Michael, and Geiser, Kenneth, "Techniques in Toxics Use Reduction," *New Solutions,* Fall 1991, pp. 25-38, and the works cited in that article. In addition to prevention and control, there is also environmental remediation, e.g., the clean-up of contaminated sites. This third option is also a third-best strategy, which has implications for occupational health.

24. Commoner, op. cit., Chapters 2. and 3.

25. Total Enclosure results in Zero Exposure to the hazard. However, the notion of Zero Exposure in occupational health is far less well entrenched than the notion of Zero Discharge or Zero Emission in environmental protection. This is another consequence of the relative isolation of occupational health from the mainstream.

26. A milestone in this process was the publication in 1971 of *Work is Dangerous to Your Health* by Stellman, J. M., Ph.D. and Daum, S. M., M.D., which deals almost exclusively with workplace health as opposed to safety hazards.

27. This doctrine is derived from the standard medical textbooks. See e.g., Clark, Duncan W., M.D., and MacMahon, Brian, M.D., Ph.D., D.P.H. *Preventive and Community Medicine,* (2nd Edition), Little Brown & Company, Boston, 1981, p. 8, where there is clearly some nervousness about the pertinence of the distinctions between prevention, intervention (treatment), and control.

28. Commoner, op. cit., pp. 76-78, clearly separates science from policy and argues that the term "science policy" is contradictory. When we are arguing the proper relationship between science and policy, it is by no means clear that we have to "derive" our policy from science. This is not the same as appealing to science in constructing policy, which is always an option.

29. See, e.g., *United Nations General Assembly,* documentation for the UNCED Conference in Brazil, 1992; Document A/CONF.151/PC/Add. 13, 20 January 1992, *Strengthening the Role of Major Groups* (Section III, Chapters 1 to 9 of Agenda 21).

30. Gordon Atherley, M.D., has suggested in conversation that holding a medical degree can be a hindrance rather than a help in the (progressive) practice of occupational health. On the other hand, I am grateful to Barry Castleman, Sc.D., for pointing out that it is impossible (to say the least) to dispense with the discipline of occupational medicine when promoting industrial health.

CHAPTER 4

Pesticide Reduction:
A Case Study From Canada

The CANADIAN federal government completed a review in 1991 of the pesticide registration process, which is the procedure by which pesticides are licensed and re-licensed for use in Canada. The review took the form of a "roundtable" with all the interested parties represented—labor, chemical producers, farmers, consumers, the medical profession, and representatives of the environmental movement.

The Canadian Labour Congress (CLC) and the Canadian Farmworkers' Union (CPU) participated because, in the wake of the American ban on Alar, it seemed that public opinion had so shifted that a major change in pesticide policy was quite a likely outcome of the project. I was involved as the Environment Representative for the CLC.

The prospects for the review were otherwise not good. There was no particular drift of policy over pesticides on the part of the federal government, which had no special desire for change and seemed to want its entire policy determined by the report of the review. Moreover, the CLC could not get any commitment from the federal Minister of Agriculture, Don Mazankowski, that the government would actually implement any consensus plan that the review might reach. Nor could we persuade the review Chair to accord full status on the review to the Canadian provincial governments, since they are responsible in practice for most of the conditions under which workers have to use toxic pesticides on farms and in many other workplaces. The federal government, for its part, was in theory a facilitator, bringing the parties together in what is known in the United States as an exercise in "interest group liberalism." In practice, the Chair of the review introduced his own proposals at a late stage of the review and they were adopted in the report as a consensus on the part of most of its members.

The CLC declined to sign the report. For one thing, we had misjudged the impact of public opinion on pesticide use (much as business managed to orchestrate the defeat of Big Green in California). The moral of the story is that without the sponsoring government's prior commitment to legislate a progressive policy, "multi-stakeholder" or "interest group" exercises are not likely to be successful. American environmentalists are accused of having fallen into the same trap, resulting in agreements which are arguably weaker than what governments would have implemented unilaterally, of their own accord. The nitrogen oxide (NOx) provisions of the acid rain controls in the new American Clean Air Act are a case in point.

A few good things came out of the review: an extension of the workplace right-to-know about pesticides, and a recommendation to set up an agency within the federal government to set targets and work plans to reduce the use of chemical pesticides in each sector across the country; but this scheme will not be enforced in regulations, and the pesticide registration system remains virtually intact.

THE ISSUES

The CLC's position throughout the review was that there should be a phasing out by 1998 of chemical pesticides for which there is significant evidence of chronic human health effects or persistent harmful effects on the environment.

"Chronic effect" means an effect on health which persists after exposure to the hazard has ceased. With pesticides and their effects on workers, communities, consumers, and wildlife, this means principally cancer, cell mutations (more or less irreversible biological changes), effects on the reproductive system and teratogenicity (effects on the unborn offspring), all very serious and often incurable. "Acute" effects, on the other hand, are those effects (except for imme-diate death from pesticide poisoning) which go away once exposure to the hazard has ceased. Acute effects can result in a lifetime of misery for workers, for example, headaches, tiredness, and skin irritations; but, apart from pesticide poisoning, they do not usually result in gross family tragedies.

The CLC certainly wanted those pesticides which posed an intolerable acute health hazard to workers banned, but the emphasis on chronic health effects still needs some explanation. Most of the acute effects, including the deaths of workers and their families, are due to employers' neglect of the elementary principles of industrial hygiene. Chronic effects, on the other hand, pose an intrinsic hazard to workers, bystanders, and the consuming public alike. No amount of control measures will eliminate the hazard.

Big Green in California was a bit different. Big Green would have eliminated, by 1996, chemical pesticides which were carcinogenic or which posed a repro-ductive hazard to human beings. In other words, Big Green limited its concern about chronic health effects to the two most notorious ones.

Either way, the dilemma is the same: in order to decide which pesticides to ban, we have to have criteria by which some pesticides will pass the test and others will fail as too dangerous to be used. We have to explain what we mean by "significant evidence" of chronic health hazards. More generally, the CLC claimed that without such legislated criteria, a pesticide control program cannot be effective. "Targets for reduction" permit too much flexibility, too many loopholes. And without criteria, we will not know whether such programs really reduce the hazards. There is no point in a 50 percent reduction in the use of pesticides if the remaining 50 percent are the most dangerous.

This dilemma has crossed journal pages before since it is part of a more general issue in toxics use reduction (TUR) programs: if under the program, X is substituted for Y, then there have to be clear and consistent criteria by which X is less hazardous or less dangerous than Y.

In the current Canadian Pest Control Products Act (PCPA) and Regulations (PCPR), there are some general references to the "safety, merit, and value" of pest control products. The Minister (that is, the Department of Agriculture) may refuse a registration if there is an "unacceptable risk of harm" to people or the environment. But the meaning of unacceptable risk is not spelled out; the PCPA is not a risk-benefit statute. One pseudo-scientific and permissive route to registration is ruled out.

This is little consolation. The act lays down no concrete criteria whereby registration must be refused and, in fact, there is no known case of a product ever having been refused registration. No doubt, there have been informal negotiations between the registration authorities and manufacturers who use the negotiations and the tentative submission of data to get a sense about whether a product will be approved or not. Alternatively, they can get an idea about whether the restrictions on use will be so severe as to turn the product into a liability rather than a business asset worth selling to the public (farmers in particular). Even if this is so, it is impossible to discern any policy on the part of the registration agency. What probably happens much more often is that an initial battery of tests reveals to a manufacturer that the company is producing a highly lethal toxin and the development of the product is not pursued.

REGISTRATION ASSURED

So far as the registration authority is concerned, the plain fact is that, provided a manufacturer submits enough data, registration is virtually assured. The PCPA does not regulate pesticides; it merely monitors their introduction into the Canadian environment. This situation will not change as a result of the Pesticide Registration Review. The final report contains a strident declaration that products which pose an unacceptable risk of harm will not be registered; but this merely reiterates the *status quo*. When the report talks about criteria for registration, it merely gives the list of registration considerations from Section 9(2) of the PCPR. Considerations are not the same as criteria. A consideration is what the registration agency has to take into account when coming to a decision. "Consideration" can mean merely consider then ignore. Criteria, on the other hand, are tests which the product must pass in order to be registered. If a product does not meet one or more criteria, it will fail and registration will be declined.

When the report talks about data requirements, it merely repeats a checklist of test topics or types of tests—or "endpoints," which are what certain tests are aimed at doing. The checklist was never legislated, nor will it be as a result of the review. Nor is it clear from such a checklist exactly what data a pesticide manufacturer has to submit, that is, what exactly would be enough to satisfy the registration authority. A legislated schedule of toxicity tests, on the other hand, would spell out exactly which tests a manufacturer has to carry out, and the manner of doing so, together with evidence that the tests were conducted properly.

The final report does contain a provision whereby the public has access to registration information before a registration decision is made so that (in theory) we do not have to wait until a product has been used and the damage done, as happened, for example, with the cancellation of the registration of Alachlor.

The first step is that the regulatory agency may ("may," not "must") publish a Proposed Regulatory Decision Document (PRDD). Then a member of the public who wants access to registration information must sign a Confidentiality Undertaking with the manufacturer. Since such agreements are essentially voluntary, it is not clear how much information, will, in fact, be divulged. Breach of the Undertaking may result in both civil and criminal penalties.

How a member of the public will be able to use such information is even less clear. Without concrete criteria in the act, there will be no way of arguing that the proposed regulatory decision is at odds with the hazard information acquired by the public under the proposed new provisions of the PCPA. In other words, the person contesting a proposed regulatory decision will have no ammunition with which to prove that the product should not be licensed under the act. For those who see access to information as a fundamental human right, the pre-registration access to information represents progress. For those who see information as a tool by which we can influence public policy, the new rights proposed in the Pesticide Registration Review are unlikely to be of much practical use. There are hundreds of new pest control products coming onto the market every year. The proposed new rules for pre-decision access to information will, at best, prevent the registration of a handful of products.

The current kinds of criteria which could be used in registration decisions are systematically inadequate to do the job. For instance, if a chemical is on an existing list of known or potential human carcinogens, this again will cut out a relatively small number of human health hazards. Usually, there is a time lag between the first use of a chronically dangerous product and the appearance of a few such products on the lists that are in current international use.

A similar argument applies to the idea of banning chemicals on the basis of clinical or epidemiological evidence. Clinical evidence is evidence that comes from doctors: an example is the observation by doctors of a rare form of liver cancer contracted by workers in vinyl chloride plants. Epidemiological evidence is statistical evidence showing an association between types of work or types of hazard on one side and rates of occupational disease on the other. Only a few chemicals would be ruled out by using these types of evidence. "Human evidence" of these sorts is always systematically behind the times. These methods always produce evidence after the damage to health has been done, that is, after a registration has been made and the product has been used for many years. Further, they only remedy a fraction of the damage. There are simply too many chemicals in use to do proper epidemiological studies on all of them. Finally, most epidemiological studies are inconclusive and controversial. There are simply too many confounding factors to point conclusively to the definitive risks posed by pesticides for epidemiology to be much use in setting an effective regulatory policy. We have to look at different methods of setting criteria for permitting or refusing registration. These methods will be concerned with estimating hazard, not calculating risk.

HOW TO DO IT RIGHT

There are, in fact, at least two alternative methods of arriving at criteria, both of which should be explored. The first is to look at the totality of toxicity data and devise a weighting system in which a chemical that gets more than a certain number of points will be banned. For instance, one of the items of toxicity data is the Lethal Dose (LD). The LD 50 is the amount of the chemical compared to body weight that will kill 50 percent of a batch of test animals. The lower the LD figure, the more dangerous the chemical, since a relatively small amount will kill a relatively large number of rats. So a low LD figure would rake up a large number of points.

But the weighting awarded to LD would be low (light) in relation to other data, since the ingestion route (swallowing the poison) is not a prime concern in industrial toxicology. Workers and their families have been killed by pesticide poisoning; but these deaths are really preventable and they are few in comparison with deaths from pesticide-induced cancer. This is the message of the United Farmworkers of America in its video, *The Wrath of Grapes*. In any case, the role of the LD in industrial toxicology has never been clear: We may have to poison a very limited number of rats in order to test drugs for human consumption, but industrial chemicals are not drugs. They are not meant to be ingested. And there may be other ways of performing tests for acute toxicity that do not involve cruelty to animals.

The part played by Lethal Concentration (LC) is a bit different. LC refers to the concentration of the vapor of the chemical and it is important because most of the hazards to pesticide workers are due to inhalation and skin absorption of the vaporized mists when they are sprayed on crops or weeds. So LC would get a higher rating than LD in the proposed weighting system.

But both LD and LC would get a relatively low weight in relation to the results of tests for chronic health hazards. For instance, acute effects are of virtually no importance to consumers who ingest pesticide residues on food, though there have been a few cases of acute poisoning of consumers, again through gross neglect of quality control at the harvesting and packaging stages. But chronic effects are very important, for example, the effects on children of apples and juice laced with Alar. Similarly, the effects of pesticides on the environment would not be so bad if wildlife were destroyed only on immediate contact with pesticides. But pesticides also typically persist, doing long-term damage to ecosystems and water supplies. All these factors should be taken into account when devising a weighting system.

The second method (proposed by the CLC in our original position paper) is to devise limits whereby a product which steps over the line in one or more tests, is automatically a candidate for banning or phasing out (that is, refusing registration). The CLC suggested, for instance, that positive results in two out of four strategically selected mutagenicity tests should qualify the test substance as a chronic human health hazard and, therefore, it should not be registered. These tests are short-term rapid-screening laboratory tests and they provide a useful method of screening out most of the real worst substances. We sometimes hear the complaint that they are less reliable than animal tests for chronic health effects (for example, carcinogenicity); but animal tests too are less than totally reliable and they too involve assumptions in applying the results of lab tests to real live human beings.

Another useful criterion is measuring a pesticide's persistence in the environment. For instance, a chemical could be phased out if the bioaccumulation factor (BCF) were greater than a certain size.

There are several important observations to be made about criteria. The first is that we are not devising a scientific scheme which can objectively compare like with like, for example, the toxicity of methyl alcohol (wood spirit, a killer) with ethyl alcohol (in booze, also a killer, but in much larger doses). Scientists who reviewed such a scheme might well regard the whole thing as garbage. This is not the point. The point is that we have to have a rough-and-ready practical scheme which does an effective job to ensure that the worst pesticides are progressively taken off the market. A lot of thought will have to go into the scheme; but it must be a practical scheme for a practical purpose, not a scientific scheme contributing to objective knowledge. The demand for "objective knowledge" has almost always been bad for workers since the continuous lack of it has meant business as usual and continued high exposure to chemicals and radiations which we know are hazardous. Constructing criteria is a job for technicians who know where they want to go, not for scientists who know what they want to know.

But whatever we decide to do, we clearly have to devise criteria which are rational (they make sense), which are consistently applied (they are fair to manufacturers), and which do a job (they get rid of gross poisons from the human environment). They do not have to be infallible. In fact, the criteria could still be revised or overturned by epidemiological or clinical evidence. Scientists will see this fault in the criteria: they are not "objective" in the sense of being perfectly well founded or perfectly reliable [1]. But this is really another way of saying that we should do nothing until we are perfectly certain of the hazard. It is another recipe for inaction, for using uncertainty as an excuse not to regulate. It is another version of the "innocent-'til-proved-guilty" version of chemical prevention and control, which is no more or less scientific than the opposite view ("guilty-'til-proved-innocent") which is being advocated here. The debate is about practical policy, not science.

In fact, there is more coherence in the attempt to devise criteria than there is in the current regulatory scheme, which in Canada (and no doubt in the United States) is haphazard and arbitrary. The current schemes cannot reduce dependency on chemical pesticides; they were never designed to do so. The best that the current scheme can do is to come out with the one-in-a-million cancer risk (risk, not hazard, again) which is a way of telling the public that all the evidence of hazard presented in the form of toxicity data really is not evidence at all. The risk calculations are a solemn and "scientific" excuse for inaction. Some people would call this a proper basis for public policy. Others would call it witchcraft.

REFERENCE

1. For the view that devising criteria for registration and control purposes is a political, pragmatic business and not a matter for scientists or for scientific decision, see for example D. Bennett, "Workplace Health and Safety: A Case Study in Union Education," *The Industrial Tutor, (U.K.), 4*:10, Autumn 1989. The most effective polemic against "science policy" is to be found, as usual, in Barry Commoner, *Making Peace with the Planet,* Pantheon Books, New York, 1990, pp. 70-78.

PART III

Pollution Prevention in Occupational Health and Environment

CHAPTER 5

The Canadian Labour Congress' Pollution Prevention Strategy

The National Environment Committee of the Canadian Labour Congress (C.L.C.) is comprised of union representatives from both public and private sectors across Canada. The committee was set up in 1987 as a subcommittee of the C.L.C. Workplace Health and Safety Committee and became a full standing committee of the C.L.C. in 1990.

From the start, the C.L.C. was committed to fighting environmental issues in close cooperation with industrial health issues. For instance, the C.L.C. Pollution Prevention Strategy is aimed at fighting a single hazard (pollution) which harms workers, communities, and the physical environment, albeit in somewhat different ways and to differing degrees.

Secondly, we were committed to working as closely as possible with national and regional environmental groups. Nearly all of the national environmental organizations are represented on the C.L.C. Environmental Liaison Group. All of the meetings of the C.L.C. Environment Committee are open to environmentalists all of the C.L.C.'s strategies and communications are openly shared. The C.L.C. works on pollution prevention as part of a caucus which includes Pollution Probe, Great Lakes United, and the West Coast Environmental Law Association.

The C.L.C. has developed a comprehensive range of education programs and policy positions on the environment (including Workers' Environmental Rights which are listed, in connection with pollution prevention, later in this chapter).

THE PRIMACY OF PREVENTION

The C.L.C.'s National Pollution Prevention Strategy (N.P.P.S.) [1] is a comprehensive program designed to eliminate pollution from Canada by the year 2000. The program emphasizes the prevention of pollution and waste at the expense of control methods once pollution has been produced by industrial activity. This distinction between prevention and control is by now well-established [2]. Pollution prevention aims at stopping pollutants from being produced, usually by banning the use of specified toxic chemicals whose transformation in workplaces results in pollution and waste or by using industrial chemicals in such a way that toxic waste is eliminated or drastically reduced. The latter method involves changes at the heart of industrial processes (and not, as with control measures, at their peripheries).

Control methods, on the other hand, are aimed at reducing pollution once pollutants have been produced by an industrial enterprise. Traditionally, they comprise:

1. The *capture* and subsequent storage of pollutants;
2. *Filtration*, whereby airborne or waterborne pollutants are removed from the waste stream by physical methods such as meshes, filters, and other permeable barriers (such as coke);
3. *Precipitation*, whereby the pollutant is chemically precipitated and then captured in its transformed state or captured by physical methods such as an electrostatic charge;
4. *Neutralization*, whereby pollutants are transformed chemically into substances which are less harmful; or (safe) destruction;
5. *Dilution*, whereby the pollutant is diluted in order to lessen its effects on anyone organism or on an ecosystem; or concentration (similar purpose);
6. *Evaporation* or *dissolution*, for example, dissolving a gas in water; or state-changes generally;
7. *Utilization*, for example, transforming a pollutant into a potentially useful (though not necessarily less toxic) product such as sulphur dioxide into sulphuric acid or using solid waste as hard core or road bed; and
8. Out-of-process *recycling*.

The characteristic of these methods is that they are inefficient in reducing pollution; they are rarely 100 percent effective and they often involve a high "energy penalty" as the cost of efficacious pollution control. For instance, dilution is effective as a method of reducing the effects of pollution on local communities (as it did when Inca built the high Superstack at Sudbury, Ontario); but the net damage to outlying communities and the environment is only mitigated if there is some well-founded scientific theory of a "threshold" of damage to living organisms. In other words, there has to be a theory that organisms can tolerate low "doses" of the pollutant, in this case, smelter emissions. Such theories are often held in the form of assumptions but, while they are plausible, they are rarely well-founded. Nor would such theories nullify the objection that smelter gases form part of the cumulative effect on the environment of other pollutants or a synergistic effect, whereby the deleterious effect is multiplied beyond the mere one-to-one unit effect of the pollutant in question.

Again, control methods often transpose the problem from one place to another, for example, from the end of the waste pipe to the storage dump or from air to water, when the pollutant is dissolved. The latter transformations are known as "media shift" [3].

ENVIRONMENTAL PROTECTION AND ECONOMICS

The first characteristic of the C.L.C. strategy is the primacy of prevention. The second characteristic is that it is a prevention strategy aimed at transforming workplaces, not at closing them down. While workers had been fighting workplace pollution long before environmental pollution first became a major public issue during the 1960s, much of the current war on pollution has been fought by the environmental movement. Some environmentalists were tempted to campaign for the closure of polluting industries, partly for the obvious reason that if a plant is not there, it cannot pollute. But there was a further reason: environmentalism was a "single-issue movement" in which other concerns, such as the creation of wealth and employment, were secondary or not on the agenda at all.

The situation is now much more constructive. The labor movement has come to regard environmental protection as a social value just as important, say, as community health and monetary benefits. The environmental movement, such as Greenpeace in Canada, has openly stated that workers' concerns and worker activism must form part of an effective grassroots environmental campaign.

Environmentalists are much more likely to succeed in alliance with workers if they adopt a "clean-up" strategy, even though a workplace pollution prevention program may not result in immediate 100 percent clean-up. There have been tangible moves of this sort in Canada at the Port Alberni pulp mill in British Columbia, at the Cominco smelter complex at Trail, B.C., at Inco in Sudbury, in the auto industry in Windsor, Ontario, and over chemical pesticide spraying of forests in New Brunswick. The number of worker environmental activists in Canada has also increased, merging the older divisions between workers and environmentalists.

Canada has just as much a problem with "de-industrialization," the decay of productive industries, as it does with industrial pollution. Strategies which recognize this fact are likely to be much more effective and successful than ones which simply demand that the problem go away. In other words, the labor movement has an industrial policy as well as an environmental policy which we want, as far as possible, to reconcile.

In general, what the C.L.C. is trying to do is to construct a pollution prevention program which depends, as far as feasible, on scientific estimates of hazards and pollution prevention priorities. But there is then a second question concerning the social-economic effects of pollution prevention measures. Thus, if we came out with a scheme which attacks the worst pollutants first, there may be reasons why the timetable for action and the scientific priorities have to be modified.

For instance, British Columbia's new rules for pulp mill effluent require a standard of a maximum of 1.5 kg of organochlorine waste per ton of pulp produced by 1995 and zero by the year 2002. But plants can get a waiver on the 1995 deadline if they attain zero by 2000. In this case, the final deadline of 2002 is not compromised; but firms are allowed flexibility in meeting it. This is exactly how things should be: tight deadlines and flexible interim targets. The difficulty from a regulatory point of view is one of ensuring that flexibility does not turn into inaction, thus in effect, compromising the final deadline when it arrives.

The pollution prevention strategy is not so much a radical position for workers as a risky one. We know from the experience of Eastern Europe that technological stagnation results in gross pollution, energy inefficiency [4], appalling effects on human health and, finally, in the death of the industrial enterprise, throwing workers out of their jobs. But technological efficiency also carries risks. Workers tend to attain longer-term job security and (sometimes) the increased benefits of higher plant productivity in the event of technological improvement; but almost always at the price of fewer jobs. This has led the C.L.C. to call, as a matter of policy and of workers' rights, for "transition measures" to protect workers in the event of environmental layoff, either because workplaces do not, in practice, meet tighter environmental protection standards (and are therefore shut down) or because new environmental technology leads to reduced work. These "transition measures" are in the form of a compensation and retraining package [5].

HEALTH, SAFETY, AND ENVIRONMENT

A third characteristic of the C.L.C. strategy is that it calls for equal treatment of pollution within the workplace as pollution (usually the same pollution) outside it—in the community and the physical environment. Again, environmentalists have sometimes failed to grasp the fact that some of the worst effects of pollution on human health occur in the work environment. This has resulted in a double standard whereby workers are officially allowed to suffer more pollution than the general public [6].

As part of a prevention plan, employers would be required to address workplace pollution equally with outside pollution, even though there may be some temporary discrepancy over who benefits most from pollution prevention measures. If the strategy is successful, workplace exposure limits [7] eventually would become redundant as the elimination of pollution becomes 100 percent effective. Further, Toxics Use Reduction (T.U.R.) programs would be assessed on the basis equally of their effects both on the work environment and on waste reduction [8].

ELEMENTS OF THE C.L.C. STRATEGY

The C.L.C. strategy has four main elements:

(i) Zero discharge as the aim of pollution prevention;

(ii) Toxics use reduction (T.U.R.) as one central tool and route to zero discharge;

(iii) Workers' Environmental Rights to entrench workers in the process of attaining the aims of pollution prevention; and

(iv) The requirement on employers to produce workplace Prevention and Control Plans (P.P.C.P.) to monitor and to ensure progress toward zero discharge.

ZERO DISCHARGE

Zero discharge of pollutants has several meanings which ought, as far as possible, to be distinguished:

(a) Banning, Severely Restricting, or Phasing Out of Dangerous Pollutants

This could equally well be called the Theory of Absolute Zero Discharge because, if a chemical is not there, it cannot pollute. The principle of banning certain chemicals, either because they are too dangerous to be used or because it is impossible to control them (or their wastes) adequately, is well established.

So far, the banning of chemicals has taken place on a case-by-case basis, often through court action, for example, the banning of the pesticide Alachlor. Criteria for banning and substitution, which need to be developed, should apply equally to the process of introducing new chemicals into industrial use, so that the function of phasing out specified chemicals is not nullified by introducing more or equally dangerous chemicals into the working or the community environment. In addition to "sunsetting" chemicals, there has to be a parallel program to prevent the increase of the "toxic burden" of the earth and "further overall loading" of the environment. There has to be provision for the "sunrising" as well as the "sunsetting" of chemicals.

(b) Virtual Elimination of Pollutants

Virtual elimination means that, by a combination or selection of production processes and end-of-pipe emission controls, pollution is radically or drastically reduced. Sometimes the standard is "no detectable level" of the pollutant. This does not preclude the possibility that ever more sensitive detection methods will later confirm the presence of the pollutant. At other times, traces of pollutants of low toxicity, for example, with rapid degradation, are permitted to come under the scope of "virtual elimination." For instance, traces of sodium chloride (common salt) solution, the result of a chlorine-related production process, would be regarded as compatible with virtual elimination, provided the effects on marine life (among other things) were negligible.

We should be clear what the aim of virtual elimination really is. The aim is to protect the environment virtually to the standard of 100 percent. For instance, traces of contaminants could continue to pollute the Great Lakes. But they should not be such as to curtail or restrict what used to be regarded as normal human activity, such as drinking the water, swimming in it, and eating the fish. At present, such restrictions, for example, on swimming or on pregnant women eating the fish, are so ominous as to deter the reasonable person from doing such things—at all, and at all times. These situations are what virtual elimination is designed to avoid, at least as regards to future pollution as opposed to the vast amount of pollution already nascent in the Great Lakes ecosystem [9].

(c) Closed-Loop Processes

The idea of a closed-loop process is that there are no discharges of any sort into the environment. The parallel within the workplace (long established) is total isolation of the production process from the work force, thus resulting in zero exposure (zero exposure to carcinogens has been C.L.C. policy since 1984). Taken literally—which we have to do in order to distinguish closed loop from virtual elimination—closed loop means that there are no emissions into the workplace or into the outside environment, not even waste water into surface water or carbon dioxide (not strictly toxic) into the atmosphere. This means that wastes have to be captured and disposed of safely and not, for example, incinerated with the consequent production of toxic air emissions and toxic ash. While such closed-loop processes are often energy efficient, using co-generation techniques, there will be a high "energy penalty" associated with the safe disposal of toxic wastes, thus indicating that there are limits to how far industrial societies can be environmentally friendly.

Even with a closed-loop process, there is still the possibility of the system breaking down, resulting in worker exposure, leaks, and spills into the outside environment or industrial disaster. Short of closing down an industrial process completely, without substitution, there are no completely fail-safe systems. Nonetheless, the closed-loop system is a practical ideal, superior to virtual elimination. Canadian research on pulp mill technology is close in theory to a closed-loop system.

TOXICS USE REDUCTION

T.U.R. is the name given to new legislative initiatives aimed at reducing the use (and thus the production) of toxic substances at the source, in several U.S. states. As such, T.U.R. is a subset of pollution prevention measures (versus pollution control) [10].The most effective is likely to be that of the Common-wealth of Massachusetts. While toxicology plays a leading role in determining the content of the Massachusetts T.U.R. program, the main stress in the program is on engineering solutions and technological development. The thrust of T.U.R. is to move governments away from risk analysis and tolerance levels for individual chemicals, toward progressive, practical prevention measures and the goal of zero discharge.

The prime aim of T.U.R. legislation is to reduce toxic discharges into the environment by means different from traditional "end-of-pipe" controls; but T.U.R. legislation can also be framed so that it embraces both worker exposure and environment-oriented requirements. Here is an example of what has been achieved and the sort of aim that is to be required in Canadian T.U.R. legislation.

Process Reformulation in Paint Stripping

> At the aircraft maintenance facilities at Hill Air Force Base in Ogden, Utah, methylene chloride-based paint strippers have been replaced by a pellet-blasting technology that removes old paint from aircraft fuselages without requiring the use of solvents. The new technology, called plastic media blasting, involves blasting the old paint surfaces with fine polymer beads shot from a high-pressure air gun. The paint chips and beads are vacuumed back to the air gun, where the beads are separated from the chips and recycled into further casting. The dry paint chips are collected and removed as a powdered waste. Not only does the process eliminate large columns of messy solvent and paint sludge, but also, it eliminates solvent air emissions and worker exposures.—Evanoff, S. P. "Hazardous Waste Reduction in the Aerospace Industry," *Chemical Engineering Progress,* April 1990.

However, we see a Canadian T.U.R. scheme differing from the Massachusetts model in a number of ways. First, the administration and enforcement of American T.U.R. laws are often weak. Some of them have provisions enabling the public to sue violators of T.U.R. law and for suing the government to ensure that T.U.R. law is observed. Canada has a different political culture from the United States. Accordingly, the C.L.C. has not strongly supported legalistic solutions to the problem of compliance. Instead, we argue for a system of administrative penalty assessments in the event of noncompliance, which complements the system of levies on chemical use. Court action as a solution has not found great favor in Canada and, rather than jailing executives, we would prefer to see a system which is effective in requiring employers to clean up their act, a pragmatic, rather than a retributive, scheme.

Secondly, we see no lower threshold limit on the use of chemicals, which would exempt an industrial enterprise from the requirements of T.U.R. One possible criticism of the Massachusetts T.U.R. scheme is that an employer could evade the requirements of T.U.R. by substituting a chemical of lower volume but higher toxicity for one of higher volume but lower toxicity, thus aggravating the problem while avoiding the T.U.R. law. One clue to this possible danger comes from the way that employers search Material Safety Data Sheets (M.S.D.S.). databases, not to acquire environmental information from them but to find cheaper and more efficacious products.

WORKERS' ENVIRONMENTAL RIGHTS

A third element in the C.L.C.'s program consists of workers' environmental rights as they relate (in this context) to the success of pollution prevention measures. Workers' environmental rights have been discussed in Canada as part of a broader program such as the idea of an Environmental Bill of Rights. However, workers' environmental rights have actually been established, to a greater or lesser degree, in the environmental protection acts of the Yukon, the Northwest Territories, Ontario, and (effectively for federal government employees only) under Section 37 of the Canadian Environmental Protection Act (C.E.P.A.).

The environmental rights, specifically, of workers are:

1. *The Right to Joint Union-Management Environment Committees.* This is sometimes called the right to participate. Provincial law should institute the right to join environment committees with rights, functions, and authority equivalent to those of the joint health and safety committee. Specific environmental powers should include the right to participate in workplace environmental audits (comprehensive audits would be required by law) and the right to participate in the framing of Pollution Prevention and Control Programs (P.P.C.P.s) (of which the T.U.R. plan forms a part). Worker members of the committee should have the right to register objections to the P.P.C.P./T.U.R. plans to the government. Legislation should provide that, where workers and management agree, the joint environment committee may be amalgamated with the joint health and safety committee, with an expanded. mandate.

2. *Whistle-Blower Protection.* This is the right of workers to divulge information to the public, the media, or to the government which concerns pollution, excessive use of energy, or waste of natural resources on the part of an employer. It is a flouting of the so-called right to manage and it overrides any supposed duty of loyalty to an employer. Several jurisdictions protect whistle-blowers to some degree; even the most progressive (the Yukon) does not accord an unqualified right.

In law, the right should be unqualified and there should be entirely adequate remedies in the event of breach of the law, for example, full reinstatement with pay, and a penalty, enough to deter, placed on employers who violate the right.

At present, most jurisdictions protect the right only partially and indirectly, through grievance arbitration. This is uncertain and unsatisfactory. While some

Canadian arbitrators have upheld the right to blow the whistle, they have not done so unconditionally. Broadly (and generalization is risky),

(i) the whistle-blower must have the best of intentions, for example, she/he must have the public interest at heart;

(ii) she/he must have grounds for believing that the employer has done something wrong, for example, a gross breach of environmental law;

(iii) she/he must give the employer the opportunity to correct the violation; and

(iv) she/he must consider the manner and tone of the whistle-blowing.

Similarly, when unions have tried to negotiate whistle-blowing in collective bargaining, they have found that employers are granting the "right," but only with the employer's "permission." Clearly, whistle-blowing has to be put into law, with full legal protection and effective redress in the event of an employer taking sanctions [11].

3. *The Legal Right to Refuse to Pollute.* The legal right to refuse to pollute is parallel to, and an extension of, the legal right to refuse unsafe work. For instance, most right-to-refuse laws in Canada require that the work hazard be, in some way, abnormal or unusual, for example, imminent danger, to justify stopping work. More generally, all the issues which we face in health and safety, such as the representative or the collective right to refuse, and payment of wages and benefits in the event of stoppage, will apply to the right to refuse to pollute. In the case of pollution, there is an even stronger case to be made that the employer should not be able to offer the job of polluting to another employee until the outcome of the case has been determined. The reason is that unsafe work sometimes has an aspect involving a degree of training and consequent responsibility, for example, the refusal to operate a fork lift without proper training. But, pollution is pollution, irrespective of who is required to carry out the act.

No government will put into effect a rule that allows work stoppage over any amount of pollution, however small. Even the progressive Yukon legislation does not go this far. A more likely result is to allow work stoppage when the worker has reason to believe that the pollution is illegal, reckless, deliberate, or in excess of the norm for the enterprise.

4. *The Right to Environmental Information.* Workers' environmental rights are ineffective without full prior knowledge about the nature and extent of pollution (as well as all other matters, such as energy use, which bear upon environmental protection). The joint environment committee should have access to all available information relating to pollution by an enterprise, public or private. Naturally, this right can only be effective if there are laws requiring the testing and measurement of emissions and effluent.

An essential first step is to add a new category of environmental protection information to W.H.M.I.S. Material Safety Data Sheets (M.S.D.S.): this would contain all available information or a reference to such information (including eco-toxicity) relating to the safe use and disposal of the product. (W.H.M.I.S. is the Workplace Hazardous Materials Information System, Canada's national workplace right-to-know law.)

Employers will raise the issue of trade secrets. In the case of pollutants, no trade secrecy can be justified. Even if it is true that revealing the identity of a pollutant would breach trade secrecy, the public interest has to override trade secrecy.

All these legal rights can be justified on grounds of equity—of which rights should properly be recognized in law. But, there is another, even better justification: that no N.P.P.S. can work effectively without them.

POLLUTION PREVENTION AND CONTROL PROGRAMS

The aim of the C.L.C.'s National Pollution Prevention Strategy is to achieve zero discharge of chemical pollutants in Canada by the year 2000 or within five years of the inauguration of the program, whichever comes first. As has been discussed, the purpose of zero discharge under N.P.P.S. is to provide equal protection to workers within polluting workplaces, the human communities outside them, and also the wider physical environment—soil, air, water, wildlife, and ecosystems.

The main method of achieving N.P.P.S. is to require employers to produce Pollution Prevention and Control Programs (P.P.C.P.) stating what they will do to achieve zero discharge within the deadline and the interim steps they will take en route to it. Such programs or plans have to be submitted every two years and with the participation of workers on Joint Union-Management Environment Committees. They have to be approved as meeting the aims and requirements of N.P.P.S. legislation.

The elements of such plans will be:

(i) processes which will be instituted to move toward zero discharge and which reduce both workers' exposure at the source and discharges to air, water, and soil;

(ii) toxics use reduction measures and plans;

(iii) traditional "end-of-pipe" emission controls, reducing pollutant discharges into soil, air, and water, as interim measures en route to zero discharge; and

(iv) progress reports on the degree of success in implementing previous P.P.C.P. plans.

Generally, N.P.P.S. legislation would apply to all workplaces, including offices, as defined under Occupational Health and Safety Acts. P.P.C.P. plans would be required for all industrial establishments, for example, mines, energy generation, primary production and processing facilities, manufacturing and chemical formulating establishments. For greater certainty, P.P.C.P. plans will be required in addition where the workplace:

(i) produces or uses chemicals which are subject to a numerical/occupational exposure limit;

(ii) produces or uses chemicals which are subject to a numerical emission control limit;

(iii) produces or uses chemicals which are the subject of process standards;

(iv) produces or uses chemicals in industrial (non-consumer) packaging as these are defined under W.H.M.I.S., except for offices which use industrially packaged chemicals in connection with the operation of office equipment. The net effect of these requirements will be to make pollution prevention, including T.U.R., a universal obligation, and to make the submission of P.P.C.P. plans a requirement of industrial establishments, broadly defined.

Finally, we want to develop some criteria whereby some chemicals count as less toxic than others, thus providing a firm guide about what really constitutes progress toward zero discharge. By the same token, such criteria would determine priorities for clean-up [12].

OBSTACLES

1. Canada's Record

The first obstacle to realizing the C.L.C.'s program is a general unwillingness on the part of governments to subject environmental protection to effective legislation. Canada's record to date on pollution prevention and control is poor; the country is simply not a world leader despite our reputation as a clean and progressive country.

One of the very few pieces of pollution prevention legislation is to be found in the regulations calling for the virtual elimination of specified dioxins and furans from pulp mill effluent, under the Canadian Environmental Protection Act (1988). Though the regulations do not specify how this is to be achieved, the net effect will be to require modifications to the pulp production process so that dioxins and furans are not produced and, therefore, cannot contaminate the waste. It is possible that some pulp mills, particularly in eastern Canada, will be unwilling or unable to meet these federal standards, resulting in closure and job losses.

Further, Canada has no T.U.R. program; no Canadian jurisdiction has enacted schemes like Massachusetts' or the other states with a statutory T.U.R. scheme.

Even on control measures, Canada's record is poor. The federal Clean Air Act was rolled into C.E.P.A. in 1988 and nullified: the only federal rules on air pollution are some cautious provisions on the control of international air pollution and, even then, only if the Canadian provinces do not (on paper) meet international obligations to which Canada is a party [13].

Few provinces have Clean Air Acts and the ones that do, such as Newfoundland and Saskatchewan, really only regulate ambient air quality (this is true of

Ontario's regulations, too). These acts regulate a very limited number of con-taminants and none of them requires certified reductions in the amounts of airborne pollution emitted by particular types of industrial plants. There is no equivalent to the 189 chemicals regulated under the 1990 amendments to the American Clean Air Act.

The principal legislative vehicle controlling water quality in Canada is the Fisheries Act and there are regulations governing, for example, discharges from refineries, mills, and mines. But nearly all of these are out of date and, as Canada's Auditor General has observed [14], poorly enforced. New pulp mill effluent regulations under the Fisheries Act have, unlike British Columbia, failed to regulate organochlorine discharges and there is, again unlike B.C., no target of zero discharge built into the regulations.

2. Jurisdiction Over Pollution Prevention

Jurisdiction over the environment is not defined in the Canadian Consti-tution and court cases have done little to clarify the issue. The result has been some overlap and duplication between the federal government's activities, on one side, and those of the 10 provinces and two territories, on the other. But, the main result has been a vacuum and paralysis. We clearly need a constructive definition of environmental authority, responsibility, and powers in any revised Canadian Constitution, discussions of which are currently taking place [15].

Other federal states have essentially resolved the issue, for example, the United States (by using other parts of the Constitution to define environmental authority), Spain (by a detailed definition in the country's new Constitution—1978), and Australia (by a series of court decisions).

The problem for authority over pollution prevention measures is particularly acute. Most of the requirements on employers would be in the form of arrange-ments within workplaces rather than "at the end of the pipe." But, such require-ments would then come under the scope of property and civil rights. These come under provincial jurisdiction and, unlike the situation in the United States, they result in clear provincial authority over labor relations and workplace health and safety (except in federal undertakings).

There are, thus, at least two possibilities. First, that we can get an effective, uniform national standard by federal-provincial and inter-provincial cooperation, thus, evading the question of jurisdiction and constitutional authority. The second is that the federal government asserts leadership in a national system of pollution prevention, leaving the courts to define the right distribution of authority and jurisdiction. Neither of these possibilities is satisfactory in the long run, since we need a constitutional definition of environmental authority pushing the question generally, but clearly, in the direction of the national (federal) power.

3. Canadian Business

The Canadian business "community" has, on the whole, not been rabidly anti-union nor has it been deeply hostile to social democracy. Recently, however, emboldened by the strength of Reagan-Thatcher style conservatism, Canadian business has launched an offensive in favor of free trade and against public institutions, against the government's regulatory program, and against Canada's social welfare system. The attacks on Ontario's New Democratic Party government can only be described as demented.

In the area of environmental protection, business has pushed a willing federal government in the direction of voluntary programs, to the exclusion of effective legislation and regulation. Despite all the talk of embracing sustainable development along the lines of the Brundtland Report of 1987, the business community advocates "relying on the market" to determine environmental policy, which really means business as usual and environmental change only to the extent that it is profitable.

In addition, the Canadian business community is naturally conservative— not known for innovation, gimmickry, or for using its imagination. A new and potentially radical idea such as pollution prevention is not likely to be embraced with enthusiasm. This means that the prospects of realizing a National Pollution Prevention Strategy are not good. The federal government, at last, has set up a National Pollution Prevention Initiative, with representation from the federal and provincial governments, labor, the environmental movement, and business. For this project to succeed in a timely manner, two things will have to happen. First, business will have to conform to a much higher degree of regulation than it has accepted in the past. Second, the provinces will have to coordinate their positive efforts in pollution prevention, a sort of thing which they have done, but only on occasion, in the past. If these two things do not happen, the federal government will have to assert its environmental authority, something that it has definitely not done in the past, sheltering behind what it professes to believe is its lack of legal environmental powers.

The C.L.C. is giving the project about a year to produce some definite results. The alternative is paralysis and a continuing vacuum in Canadian environmental standards. Either way, the C.L.C. will continue its program of union environmental education, coalition-building, and grass-roots worker environmental activism.

REFERENCES

1. The C.L.C. National Pollution Prevention Strategy was developed through the C.L.C. National Environment Committee, the C.L.C. National Workplace Health & Safety Committee, and the C.L.C. Toxic Substances Working Group. The strategy was endorsed by the Environment Committee (of which I am Secretary) in February 1992. Particular Canadian unionists who contributed to the development of the strategy were: Cathy Walker (C.A.W.); Brian Kohler (CEP); Cliff Andstein

(B.C.G.E.U./N.U.P.G.E.); Larry Stoffman (U.F.C.W.); Andy King (U.S.W.A.); and Jennifer Penney (O.F.L.).

2. Commoner, B. *Making Peace with the Planet.* New York: Pantheon, 1990, Chapter 3. Rossi, M., et al. "Techniques in T.U.R.," *New Solutions,* Fall, 1991, and the works cited in that article. Barry Commoner tends to confine prevention to the wholesale banning of chemical substances, confining their use to the manufacture of pharmaceuticals and videotape (two products which, ironically, we have far too much already).

3. The distinction between prevention and control is not always as absolute as it may seem. For one thing, prevention methods are not always 100 percent effective either. For instance, a chemical may be eliminated to be replaced by a substitute: but the substitute is likely to be at best less harmful than what it replaced, not 100 percent safe. The "soft" CFCs are a case in point. Even then, we have to work out a scheme by which we have reason to believe that substitutes are, in fact, less harmful than what they replace. This scientific exercise in priority-setting or criteria for relative environmental friendliness is not well advanced. The Massachusetts T.U.R. program, for instance, does not embody any scheme for rating the relative hazard of different chemicals, relying evidently on common sense for what counts as a reduction of hazard and, therefore, of the resulting waste.

Or again, take this example: A "site-specific intermediary" is a chemical compound both produced and used within a single industrial enterprise in the middle of an industrial process. If the efficiency of the industrial process is increased, the concentration of the resulting pollutant, for example, residues of the intermediary, can be reduced. This will count as a prevention method. Or, the pollutant can be controlled by anyone of the methods listed above. From the point of view of the environment, there may be little to choose between the approaches, since (cost aside) the result may be the same. Clearly, if a pollutant is treated on the way out of the waste pipe (for example, scrubbers) or at the end of the pipe (for example, secondary treatment ponds for pulp mill effluent), these will count as control methods. But, if a potential pollutant, such as the residue of a site-specific intermediary, is treated at the periphery of an industrial process, but deep within the plant, it will count as a prevention method.

This is not to say that there may not be a better prevention method such as the elimination (or substitution) of the site-specific intermediary; but there is a gray area in which the distinction between prevention and control becomes blurred. Crudely, if the method is an engineering process method, it will count as prevention. If the method depends on chemical or physical treatment of a pollutant (including a persistent site-specific intermediary), it will count as a control method.

The general point remains: prevention is primary, and it is much more effective in reducing pollution than control.

4. Cairncross, F., *Costing the Earth,* Economist Books, London: 1991, Page 110 ff, documents the energy inefficiency of East European industry.

5. Canadian Labour Congress. *C.L.C. Policy Statement on the Environment,* endorsed by the C.L.C. Executive Council, December, 1991. The C.L.C. position is in the same realm of debate as that in the United States over a Superfund for Displaced Workers. See, for example: Wykle, L., Morehouse, W., & Dembo, D., *Worker Empowerment in a Changing Economy, Jobs, Military Production and the Environment,* New York:

Apex, 1991. But, the Superfund idea seems to me to condone too readily the massive de-industrialization of the United States, something that American governments have failed to prevent over the last decade.

6. For instance, worker body burden limits for lead are several times more lax than the recommended standard for the general public. In ionizing radiation protection standards, the discrepancy between levels for workers and for the public is enormous.

7. Workplace exposure limits include Permitted Exposure Limits (PELs), Threshold Limit Values (TLVs), and the like.

8. Murray, L., "The Politics of Pollution Prevention," *New Solutions,* Fall, 1991.

9. Attacks on the idea of zero discharge take two forms:
(i) Since a discharge level of literally zero is rarely possible, short of shutting down a polluting industry, the idea of zero should be abandoned; or
(ii) Since Virtual Elimination is a radically unclear idea or incapable of a proper definition, it should be abandoned in favor of something less ambitious and more attainable.
All this is in need of an extended examination, dealing with the relationship between science and public policy and ways in which business seeks to discredit the environmental movement, ostensibly on scientific grounds.

10. Rossi et al. Cited at Note 2 above, Page 1.

11. Myers, Q. C. M. and Matthews Lemieux, V. J., "Whistle-Blowing Employee Loyalty and the Right to Criticize: The Employee's Perspective," *Labor Arbitration Year Book,* Butterworths, Canada, 1991, Volume 2.

12. Some ideas for the ranking of hazards and criteria are to be found in Bennett, D. "Pesticide Reduction, A Case Study from Canada," *New Solutions,* Fall, 1991.

13. Canadian Environmental Protection Act. Sections 61-65.

14. *Report of the Auditor General of Canada,* October, 1990.

15. See, for example, "The Environment and the Canadian Constitution, A Discussion Paper," Draft 3. C.L.C. Environment Committee, June, 1991.

CHAPTER 6

Prevention and Transition

Strategies to protect workers' health and the environment outside of the workplace, were, respectively, once based on the notion of *control*: a series of controls (engineering and administrative) in the workplace and emission controls to protect the public environment. Two parallel changes occurred. The first was a shift from the general principles of control to the notion of a hierarchy of control measures and the second was a recasting of the Hierarchy of Controls into what has been called a Hierarchy of Prevention and Controls. This chapter cites the Canadian experience to show that this twofold shift is a progressive and constructive move; the United States provides both the sources of the problem and some solutions. "Just Transition" for workers during environmental change was developed in the context of chemical bans and phase-outs. The concept is now much broader. The chapter argues that certain pollution prevention measures have been construed as an attack on workers' rights; but this problem can be resolved to the benefit of both workers' health and environmental protection. Explanation of the relation of pollution prevention to Just Transition is a part of the solution.

THE TRADITIONAL THEORY OF CONTROL

The *prevention* of health, safety, and environmental hazards is usually defined as a series of techniques or methods to *avoid the creation* of hazards. The control of hazards aims to *reduce* or *mitigate* the effects of hazards once they have been created. In the field of occupational health and safety, the discipline of industrial hygiene has two salient characteristics: first, an emphasis on control at the expense of prevention and, second, a failure to develop a hierarchy of preferred protective techniques. The consequences of these characteristics are similar: both result in a failure to adopt the most effective techniques for protecting workers' health and safety. Neither provides any pressure on employers, occupational health professionals, or on workers themselves to institute the most effective protection measures in the workplace.

Here are some examples. An early example from the U.S. National Safety Council [1] actually comes closest to a Hierarchy of Controls. Ten methods of engineering control are listed (without pretending they are exhaustive). Since substitution of a less harmful material is at the top of the list, with process alteration to "minimize worker contact" with the hazard the second, there is an indication that the list is in order of preference or effectiveness. A later publication, specifically on workplace chemical hazards, simply lists substitution and engineering controls as primary means of control, with personal protective equipment (PPE) and "administrative controls" as less desirable alternatives [2]. The bulk of the discussion is then on engineering controls.

At about the same time, another publication lists substitution as the best method, followed by engineering controls, with PPE as a distant third [3]. In a more recent example, the emphasis has shifted somewhat. Methods of control are divided into three categories: control at the source, control along the air path, and control at the receiver. It is clear that the first of these is to be preferred and the first two items listed under source control are substitution and process changes, e.g., "airless paint spraying." There is also an emphasis on the need to consult with the industrial hygiene engineer at the design stage of the facility, though this is on the grounds of cost savings rather than increased worker protection [4].

The picture does not change much in works that are specifically aimed at workers or unions. One early famous example sets down the three conventional categories of elimination of the hazard at the source, ventilation, and PPE; though there is rather more discussion of the first of these than in the industrial hygiene texts and we see, for the first time, the use of the word "elimination" rather than "control" at the source [5]. However, control measures as well as preventive or elimination methods are still put into the first of the three categories.

This categorization was taken up in a Canadian worker training manual under the heading "control measures" (see Figure 1).

Later examples of worker-oriented publications are little different. The term used is "Principles of Control" rather than a Hierarchy of Controls, though several examples include the need to protect the surrounding community as well as eliminate the hazard in the workplace [6]. As we will see, this foreshadows important developments in environmental protection.

There is a curious discrepancy between the role of prevention in industrial hygiene and in industrial medicine. The latter makes a conventional distinction between Primary, Secondary, and Tertiary Prevention, which suggests (disingenuously) that physicians are concerned solely with prevention rather than treatment and remedy. But at least we see a predilection for Primary Prevention, with the suggestion that Primary Prevention in the form of elimination of the hazard at the source should be the focus of occupational medicine [7]. The term Primary Prevention is not used in industrial hygiene and it is odd that it is used in a discipline that deals essentially with the treatment of maladies rather than the engineering disciplines which inform the elimination of workplace hazards

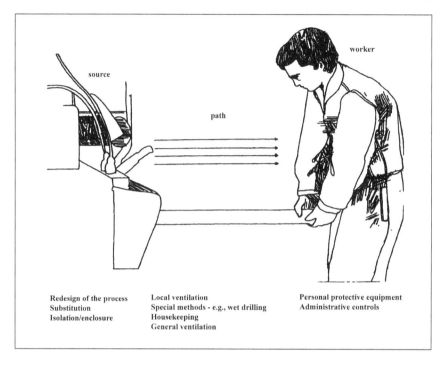

Figure 1. From *Occupational Health and Safety: A Training Manual,*
Copp Clark Pitman, Toronto, p. 46, 1982.

[8]. A further oddity is that the medical removal of workers from work hazards (e.g., the removal of workers who have been "leaded" from a lead smelter) counts as a Primary Prevention technique in medicine but receives a low ranking as an administrative control in industrial hygiene.

Turning from the work environment to environmental protection, the main focus of effort in the same period was not on prevention but on pollutant *emission controls*. Polluters were (and are) required to limit emissions of pollutants or control their flow of wastes into the environment by a number of control methods. The form of limitation on emissions varies according to the pollutant. For instance, there are: 1) simple limits on the *amount* of a pollutant, such as acid gases, that a plant may emit or release per year; or 2) limits on the *ratio* of a pollutant to product, such as pulp to pulp mill effluent; or 3) limits on the *concentration* of pollutants in emissions, such as heavy metals, or 4) *procedural rules*, e.g., for handling waste or the reporting at spills. The last of these includes indicating the technology that must be used to control pollutants, particularly water-borne pollutants.

Again, we do not see a hierarchy of environmental controls. There are rarely even lists. Table 1 was pulled together by the Canadian Labour Congress.

Table 1. Traditional Environmental Control Measures

The main methods of pollution control, in no particular order, are:

- the *capture* and subsequent storage of pollutants;
- *filtration*, whereby airborne or waterborne pollutants are moved from the waste stream by physical methods such as meshes, filters, and other permeable barriers, such as coke;
- *precipitation*, whereby the pollutant is chemically precipitated and then captured in its transformed state or captured by physical methods such as an electrostatic charge;
- *destruction*, for example incineration, or neutralization, whereby pollutants are transformed chemically or biologically into substances that are less harmful;
- *dilution*, whereby the pollutant is diluted or flushed in order to lessen its effects on any one organism or on an ecosystem; or concentration to narrow the effects of disposal;
- *evaporation* or *dissolution*—for instance, dissolving a gas in water;
- *utilization*—for example, transforming a pollutant into a potentially useful (though not necessarily less toxic) product, such as sulphur dioxide into sulphuric acid or using solid waste as hard core or road bed;
- *out-of-process recycling* (a mode of reuse) where the recycling is not an integral part of the production process;
- *media-shift*, whereby a waste-stream is diverted from one medium such as air, soil, or water, to another, on the rationale that the medium-shift makes the pollutant less harmful; and
- *state-changes*—a change to the solid, liquid, or gaseous state on the rationale that the new state is less harmful.

Source: *A Workers' Manual on Pollution Prevention*, Canadian Labour Congress, Ottawa, Canada, Appendix 8, p. 57, 1998.

In occupational health, the problem is not that there is no such concept as prevention. Rather, prevention and control are not rigidly distinguished as protective techniques.

Thus, while most sources acknowledge a rough scheme of preference among protective methods, none depicts a hierarchy and, thus, none is able to set down a hierarchy of protective measures with prevention at the top. On the contrary, prevention and control are often confused and conflated with each other. In Canada, for instance, health and safety as a discipline is often divided between what is called prevention, in contrast to the remedial side of regulatory or other activity. The remedial side includes workers' compensation, medical treatment, and rehabilitation of injured workers. The prevention side is everything else, principally control measures, most of which have nothing at all to do with prevention as initially defined in this chapter.

PREVENTION IN ENVIRONMENTAL PROTECTION

Until the late 1980s, the role of prevention in environmental protection was in an even worse state. There always was a distinction between prevention, control, and remediation of environmental hazards, with some unclarity over the terms "clean-up," abatement, and mitigation. But even here, there was (and still is) confusion, even obfuscation. This is the official definition of the Prevention of Pollution by the International Organization for Standardization (ISO):

> Use of processes, practices, materials, products or energy that avoid, reduce or control pollution, which may include recycling, treatment, process changes, control mechanisms, efficient use of resources and material substitution. [ISO 14000,3. 13]

Here, prevention, control, and remediation are mixed up together with no possibility of a hierarchy. The net result is that there is no focus on prevention as the most effective approach to environmental protection. Further, this definition allows business to claim that prevention is something they do all the time. There is, it is claimed, nothing new or different about pollution prevention.

THE REVOLT:
PREVENTION VERSUS CONTROL

Two developments seem to have occurred simultaneously. First, in Canadian labor circles at least, the term Hierarchy of Controls has come to rival the traditional Principles of Control. It is, however, hard to find written sources, such as union education materials, where the term Hierarchy of Controls is used. The motive was clear: to accord a priority to those methods that are the most efficacious in protecting workers' health. Second, prevention comes to be the key concept in protective measures, with demands, for example, for a Prevention Regulation under occupational health statutes [9]. There were some important precedents, even if the actual term "prevention" was not used. Part X of the Regulations under the Canada Labour Code (Health and Safety), which applies to workers under federal jurisdiction, has long had a "substitution rule"; hazardous substances in the workplace must be substituted with non-hazardous or less hazardous substances wherever it is reasonably practicable [x: 11].

But where did the emphasis on prevention come from? It came from pressure to protect the environment external to the workplace and, to that extent, the demand for prevention came from the environmental rather than from the labor movement. The revolt against control measures as the key to environmental protection began in the late 1980s. The key thinker and publicist of the revolt was Barry Commoner. He pointed out that the environmental control program had in 20 years been a failure. The only successes were where the pollutant or its source had been totally removed from the environment, such as airborne lead, DDT, mercury in surface waters and radioactive fallout. Thus, Barry Commoner said, in 1990:

> In sum, there is a common explanation for each of the few sharp reductions in emissions: in each case environmental degradation was **prevented** by simply stopping production or use of the pollutant. This suggests an addition to the informal environmental law: If you don't put something into the environment, it isn't there. . . . Controls yield little or no improvement in environmental quality because they are ultimately self-defeating. [10]

Out of such thinking arose a whole theory of prevention, particularly as it applied to chemical hazards. The overall umbrella concept is usually (not always) pollution prevention and it embraces a large number of concepts and practices, such as the use of processes, practices, materials, products, or energy that avoid or minimize the creation of pollutants and waste [12]; chemical bans, phase-outs ("sunsetting"), source reduction, Toxics Use Reduction (TUR) and chemical substitution [13]. The idea is to focus on prevention and to remove control and remediation entirely from the scope of environmental protection programs. Legislation followed. The Massachusetts Toxics Use Reduction Act (TURA) was enacted in 1989 and the New Jersey Pollution Prevention Act in 1991. The U.S. Pollution Prevention Act became law in 1990; the various state pollution prevention and TUR laws, passed both before and after 1990, vary widely in quality and effectiveness. The characteristic of most of these laws was that, in themselves, they eliminated the need for risk assessment as a technical device to mediate the problem and its solution, when risk assessment is seen as a permissive scientific technique that is responsible for lax prevention and control policies [14]. This has not, of course, prevented the adoption of risk assessment techniques in other environmental protection regimes.

In all this effort, health and safety lagged behind environmental protection. In the 1970s, the focus of thinking and effort shifted from physical injuries and compensation to occupational diseases and the "hidden hazards of work." But the parallel shift from control to prevention was slow in coming. The characteristic of pollution prevention is that it protects the work environment, the health of communities outside the work place, and the physical environment or ecosystems, alike. Pollution prevention connects occupational health and the environment in new and convincing ways. Yet workers, for instance, played very little part in the construction of the Massachusetts TUR Act and, unlike environmentalists, workers play no part on its advisory body. This lack of worker input has had a stultifying effect on the adoption of pollution prevention and TUR as powerful weapons in fighting occupational disease.

In some ways, the prospects for prevention in health and safety have worsened. There is now a wholesale attempt to import risk assessment techniques into health and safety decision-making and, instead of promoting prevention measures, workers are forced to spend their time fighting a technique that, far from being promoted, ought to be put into the garbage can [15].

But things are starting to change. The labor movement is beginning to adopt pollution prevention, thus in effect importing an environmental protection technique into the work environment. The Canadian Auto Workers Prevent Cancer Campaign is a prime exercise in putting prevention ahead of controls and other Canadian unions too have promoted prevention as the key to health and safety [16]. A recent International Labour Organization (ILO) draft Code of Practice [11] even refers to a "recognized hierarchy of preventive and protective measures": the reference to a hierarchy and to prevention are entirely new. In adopting pollution prevention, the labor movement has realized that we have to fundamentally change our outlook about the relationship between prevention and the more traditional Hierarchy of Controls. Thus, the Canadian Labour Congress, in its education programs, has tried to revamp the Hierarchy of Controls and replace it with the new Hierarchy of Prevention and Controls (see Figure 2) [17].

In the new hierarchy, priority is given to elimination, substitution, chemical use reduction, and closed loop systems. The new hierarchy recognizes that we still have to use traditional control measures, but it gives them a low priority in favor of the new prevention regimes developed, essentially, in connection with environmental protection.

The new hierarchy does, however, pose some problems, understandable enough when we bear in mind that it breaks new ground. Under heading #2, preventive maintenance is listed as a prevention method, yet this hardly fits with the initial definition of pollution prevention whereby prevention refers to avoidance techniques, not to the management or control of hazards once created. The latter is the obvious way of categorizing maintenance procedures. Again, in pollution prevention and TUR doctrine, closed loop methods count as pollution prevention, yet here too pollutants are created, albeit recycled inside the production process. The new hierarchy puts closed loop under heading #3, as a control method, arguably where it properly belongs. Generally, prevention and control methods are organized in the hierarchy in a pragmatic, common sense way, rather than according to strict definitions.

"JUST TRANSITION"

The movement to protect the livelihoods of workers caught up by environmental change was directly connected to pollution prevention. Progressive unions such as the Oil, Chemical and Atomic Workers International Union (OCAW) and the Communication, Energy and Paperworkers Union of Canada (CEP) recognized that their members worked in the "toxic economy" and they proposed measures that would take us out of the toxic economy, while protecting the livelihoods of the workers at the same time. The principal device for doing this was to be the creation of the Superfund for Workers, modeled on the U.S.

1. **Eliminate Toxic Substances and Processes**

   —change the product to <u>eliminate</u> toxic products
   —change the process to <u>eliminate</u> the use of toxic substances or the
   creation of toxic by-products
   —substitute non-toxic substances

2. **Reduce the Use of Toxic Substances**

   —change workplace practices to use less of a toxic substance
   —change workplace processes to use less of a toxic substance
   —preventive maintenance and modification of operations to reduce spills,
   leaks, and emissions

3. **Reduce Exposures to Toxic Substances by "Control at the Source"**

   —closed loop systems (sealed processes, in which waste is reused)
   —isolation/total enclosure of the process
   —process redesign to control more effectively

4. **Reduce Exposures by Control "Along the Path" of the Hazard**

   —separate ventilation for areas where toxic substances are handled
   —local ventilation
   —special methods, e.g., wet drilling
   —better work areas
   —general ventilation

5. **Reduce Exposures by Controls "at the Worker"**

   —personal protective equipment (PPE)
   —administrative controls, e.g., rotating workers in a dangerous job
   —medical monitoring

Figure 2. The Hierarchy of Prevention and Controls.
Source: From the CLC Health and Safety Education Course Program,
Module #7, Pollution Prevention versus Control.

environmental Superfund for the clean-up of contaminated sites. Benefits were
to be distributed along the lines of the GI Bill (1944) for returning veterans of
World War II [18].

Since the early 1990s, the concept of Just Transition has been expanded and
refined, with far more thought being given to sources of funding and far more of
an emphasis on re-employment and alternative employment on the benefit side of

the equation. Further, the *scope* of the industrial changes to which Just Transition will apply has been expanded. The changes that would result from the removal of chlorine compounds from industrial processes, the proposed treaty to address the elimination of selected organic pollutants (Persistent Organic Pollutants), and the dramatic changes that would result from effective climate change measures are all areas where the labor movement sees an application for Just Transition. The idea of Just Transition is to be applied to all areas in which the effects of environmental change on patterns of employment are likely to be deep and widespread. What began as a union response to environmental pressures is now turning, as planned, into a social movement with an environmental dimension. Support is also widening, with organizations such as the Canadian Labour Congress [19], the International Confederation of Free Trade Unions (ICFTU), and the Trade Union Advisory Council (TUAC) of the Organization for Economic Cooperation and Development (OECD) having active programs under the umbrella of Just Transition [20].

JUST TRANSITION AND POLLUTION PREVENTION

From the beginning, it was clear that Just Transition was to come into play because of plans to ban or phase out specific toxic chemicals. "This program proposes that workers who lose jobs due to international trade agreements or as a result of the environmental phase out or ban on toxic substances should suffer no net loss of income. . . . The threat [to jobs] involves banning or phasing out a toxic substance . . ." [21]. Or again: "Pollution prevention strategies can protect both workers and communities, and create jobs in existing facilities. But pollution prevention in the form of bans and phaseouts does cause long-term and massive job loss. . . . There are some real pollution prevention success stories and innovations being implemented around the country in a variety of industries" [22].

Clearly, both pollution prevention and Just Transition are important for the workers in chemical-producing industries. But there is a problem in that the linkage of the two concepts has caused them to work against each other, to the detriment of the whole labor movement. The first stage was an unfortunate choice of terminology. Instead of linking Just Transition in the first instance with the moves to ban or phase out specific industrial chemicals, it was linked instead with the whole global concept of pollution prevention. The result was that the problem for workers was seen to be *all of the components of pollution prevention*, including Toxics Use Reduction, which is of prime benefit to millions of workers in the chemical-using industries. As we have seen, pollution prevention concepts, including use reduction, are now the key factor in promoting industrial health. Attack them and you are attacking the fundamental workers' agenda for achieving a healthy work environment. Yet this is what has happened.

In 1991, Michael Merrill wrote an article entitled "No Pollution Prevention Without Income Protection: A Challenge to Environmentalists." Much of the article dealt with the relationship between chemical bans and the Superfund for Workers [23]. But Merrill also used the article to attack pollution prevention generally and TUR legislation in particular as "striking at the heart of the American economy." The unavoidable impression from the article is that workers should not support TUR programs unless there is a full-scale transition program in place such as the Superfund. Such statements from the friends of labor are not helpful because they are based on a poor appreciation of the causes of occupational disease and the value of TUR as an occupational health strategy.

What then *do* we need? Merrill and others have rightly called for labor-environmental alliances so that Just Transition forms an integral part of environmental progress. But we also have to mobilize the whole of the labor movement, particularly those working actively for TUR programs in their own workplaces, to join the campaign for Just Transition. There has to be a social contract, not only between workers and environmentalists, but within the labor movement itself. Otherwise, workers in chemical-producing industries will be induced to take part in an attack on the very programs that are of central importance in protecting workers' health from chronic diseases.

In its Just Transition policy, the Canadian Labour Congress [19], addressed this very point. The policy was constructed with the active participation of a large number of major unions from both the chemical-producing and the core using industries and from both public and private sectors. It was understood that the public sector could be affected by environmental change as deeply as private sector industries. It was further understood that workers in the chemical-producing industries needed the support of unions in the user industries for Just Transition to become an effective social program. Workers in the chemical-using industries (including the public sector) are the main beneficiaries of pollution prevention programs while the need for Just Transition in the chemical-producing industries was understood right from the beginning. Workers in the chemical-producing industries were the source of demands to turn Just Transition from a sectoral to a national program.

Endorsement of Just Transition by Canada's national environmental organizations is another matter, some welcoming the environmental commitment that Just Transition implies, others suggesting that employers will use Just Transition as a new form of condition and therefore barrier to environmental change. The alliances that the Canadian labor movement is committed to building are by no means easy for either workers or for environmentalists outside the labor movement.

REFERENCES

1. *Accident Prevention Manual for Industrial Operations*, Fifth Edition, pp. 39-36. Original Copyright 1964.
2. N. H. Proctor and J. P. Hughes, *Chemical Hazards of the Workplace,* Philadelphia and Toronto, 1978.

3. N. Irving Sax, *Dangerous Properties of Industrial Materials*, Fifth Edition, Section 1, Page 10, New York, 1979.
4. B. A. Plog (ed.), *Fundamentals of Industrial Hygiene*, Third Edition, pp. 457-458. National Safety Council, 1988 (originally published in 1971). Ironically, a contemporary example is the furthest removed from the grading of control methods in terms of preference: see *The Occupational Environment—Its Evaluation and Control*, S. P. DiNardi (ed.), Chapter 31 by D. J. Burton, pp. 829-830, American Public Health Association, 1997.
5. J. M. Stellman and S. Daum, *Work is Dangerous to Your Health,* Chapter 9, pp. 290-326, Controlling Pollution in the Workplace, New York, 1971.
6. *Occupational Health and Safety. A Training Manual*, Chapter 6, Principles of Control, published by the (Ontario) Workers' Health and Safety Centre, 1992.
7. See, e.g., D. W. Clark and B. McMahon, *Preventive and Community Medicine,* Second Edition, Little Brown & Company, Boston, p. 8, 1991.
8. These issues are discussed in D. Bennett, Occupational Health. A Discipline Out of Focus, *Journal of Public Health Policy, 14*:3, pp. 276-298, Autumn 1993.
9. In the project to amend Part II of the Canada Labour Code, the Canadian Labour Congress argued successfully for a Prevention Regulation under the revised statute.
10. B. Commoner, *Making Peace with the Planet,* Pantheon Books, New York, p. 43, 1990.
11. *Draft Code Of Practice On Safety In The Use of Synthetic Vitreous Fibre Insulation Wools,* Geneva, p. 2, 1999.
12. This is from the definition of pollution prevention by the Government of Canada in its 1995 publication *Pollution Prevention. A Federal Strategy for Action.*
13. One of the first publications pointing out the perils of confusing prevention and control was M. Rossi, M. Ellenbecker, and K. Geiser, Techniques in Toxics Use Reduction, *New Solutions, 2*:2, pp. 26-27, Fall 1991. (The authors see TUR as a subset of pollution prevention techniques.)
14. See, principally, R. Ginsburg, Quantitative Risk Assessment and The Illusion of Safety, *New Solutions, 3*:2, Winter 1993; also Risk Assessment As a Regulatory Device, two articles with the same title by D. Bennett and M. Winfield respectively, in *Regulatory Efficiency and the Role of Risk Assessment,* M. D. Mehta (ed.), Queen's University, Kingston, Ontario, 1995.
15. See F. Mirer, UAW testimony to the U.S. Senate on S. 981, The Regulatory Improvement Act, reprinted in *Great Lakes United, 12*:1, Winter/Spring 1998.
16. See The Workplace Killer: Occupational Cancer Should Be Called an Epidemic, *Outfront,* the magazine of the Canadian Labour Congress, *2*:3, Fall 1998; also the CLC National Pollution Prevention Strategy, Ottawa, 1998, an advanced version of a strategy reported in *New Solutions, 3*:3, Spring 1993.
17. The Hierarchy of Prevention and Controls was derived from an entirely original idea, *Towards A New Hierarchy of Controls,* on the part of J. Penney, a doctoral candidate in the Department of Work Environment, University of Massachusetts Lowell.
18. See *Worker Empowerment in a Changing Economy,* L. Wykle, W. Morehouse, and D. Dembo, The Apex Press, New York, 1991.
19. The Canadian Labour Congress Policy on Just Transition For Workers During Environmental Change was endorsed by the CLC Executive Council on April 29, 1999.

20. See the ICFTU-TUAC Convention Trade Union Statement to the U.N. Climate Change Convention Conference of the Parties (COP4), November 1998.
21. R. Wages, President of OCAW, *Hazards, 63,* 1998.
22. *A Just Transition For Jobs and The Environment*, produced by the Public Health Institute and the Labor Institute, New York, p. 81, 1998.
23. *New Solutions, 1*:3, Winter 1991. More clearly, R. Miller and S. J. Lewis drew transition and chemical bans together in "Orderly Transition for Chemical Sunsetting," *New Solutions, 5*:1, Fall 1994.
24. Principally, R. Kazis and R. L. Grossman in *Fear At Work,* Pilgrim Press, New York, 1982. See also the open letter from L. Leopold and S. Kieding to the editor, *New Solutions, 7*:3, Spring 1997.

PART IV

Cancer Prevention

CHAPTER 7

Cancer Battles and the Sleep of Reason: Review

OVERVIEW

Cancer Battles and the Sleep of Reason is an inquiry into the role of scientific experts in environmental health policy-making. The chapter first establishes two propositions: that there is no necessary relationship between science and environmental health policy; and that risk assessment is not the only science of environmental health. It then asks the question: why should policy-makers consult the scientific experts? If experts are to be consulted, there will have to be some way of grading experts as to the quality of their advice and their usefulness to policy-makers. A mode of grading experts is provided in *Environmental Cancer—A Political Disease?* by S. Robert Lichter and Stanley Rothman. But the arguments in this book are shown to be worthless; the book fails to address the underlying issue of why the experts should be consulted at all. The chapter concludes that experts are to be consulted whenever policy-makers consider their advice to be essential or useful. There is nothing in the scientific disciplines that entrenches them in the policy-making process; the opinions of scientific experts have no special place in environmental health policy.

ENVIRONMENTAL CANCER—A POLITICAL DISEASE? by S. Robert Lichter and Stanley Rothman, Yale University Press, 1999.

Let us suppose a group of policymakers proposed to reduce the volume of chemical pesticides released into the environment. They made it a rule that only a small, selected number of chemical pesticides were to be allowed, based solely on agricultural need. Asked to defend their stance, they said that it was not a good idea to spread chemical poisons needlessly over the human and physical environment. There were effects on agricultural productivity, to be sure, but they could be mitigated by non-chemical pest control methods. Also, we should measure agricultural output by food value in relation to depletion of soil quality, not simply by volume of product.

Those opposed to the move replied that if there were any detriments to human health, they were small compared with the agricultural benefits of the unrestricted use of pesticides. Besides, most of the human detriments could be avoided by the licensing of pesticide applicators, strict rules over spraying, and the use of personal protective equipment. No doubt, chemical pesticides degrade the environment, but here again the price is worth paying in terms of agricultural productivity. The degradation of the environment is minuscule compared with the move from wild country to agricultural settlement.

The idea of allowing only a small number of pesticides is essentially the pest control policy of Sweden, Austria, and the erstwhile German Democratic Republic.

The point of this policy debate is that it can be conducted entirely without reference to scientific expertise. Such a scenario could not easily be envisaged in the United States, not least because of the presence of a powerful business lobby representing a major manufacturing industry. More pertinent is the objection that the United States is not a parliamentary democracy and the structure of its political system is such as to rule out radical moves of this sort. It may also be true that property rights in the U.S. Constitution would prohibit discrimination over manufacturers' different products. It is bad enough that whole classes of product are taken off the market, even worse when one manufacturer's pesticide for a given set of crops is allowed, when another's pesticide, chemically different but performing the same function, is prohibited. The proposed scheme is against equity and natural justice.

The least that would have to happen is that there be some rational way of deciding which products are to be allowed and which not. There are several ways in which this could be done. The first is determining a yardstick of agricultural efficacy (how well does the pesticide work) and allowing only those above a certain threshold to qualify. But this would be so uncertain, time-consuming, variable and tenuous that it would be likely in practice to be stalled indefinitely. Enter the scientific experts.

RISK ASSESSMENT IS NOT THE ONLY SCIENCE
OF ENVIRONMENTAL HEALTH

The first reaction of most scientific experts would be to challenge the usefulness and propriety of the scheme proposed. They would offer the only tool on hand: risk assessment. Do a risk assessment on each of the candidates for approval or rejection. If a pesticide really does pose a significant risk: take it off the market. The characteristic of such assessments is that they are not based centrally on epidemiology or direct evidence of human health effects. When pesticides are first approved, there is little such evidence available and once the evidence does start to come in, it is mighty difficult to get the approval cancelled. So risk assessments are usually based on calculation from sources of non-human evidence and data. A threshold of harm also has to be established, estimated, or calculated from the data. Under this procedure, almost nothing is ruled out. Risk assessment allows pretty much every application for approval to be accepted. It could certainly not be used to provide the rationale for a radical proposal such as the one described.

Some other scientific rationale must be sought. This can be discerned from Table 1 [1].

Table 1 sets down a number of environmental and human health criteria (under "Element Name"), then assigns an Endpoint and Unit (the type of test or data to be used), then scores each candidate substance a numerical value (0-10). The scores for each candidate, i.e. each substance subjected to the scoring matrix, are then ranked in numerical order.

In theory, the scoring system is an abstract schema, that can be used for different political purposes. It could be used, for example, to determine which substances should be investigated further—such as doing epidemiological studies—on the grounds that the highest scoring substances are likely to be most detrimental in practice. Or it could be used for regulatory purposes. In fact, the Ontario Ministry of the Environment in the early 1990s used the scoring system as a basis for the development of multimedia standards and water quality guidelines for selecting chemicals of high priority for air emission control and for waste management [2]. The policy purpose in question will determine where to draw the line under the score chart: for example, if there were only limited cash available, policymakers might sponsor epidemiological studies on only the three top scorers over a certain volume of the substance in use or emitted. From the point of view of science, these lines are arbitrary. From the point of view of policy, they may be set pragmatically, e.g., how much environmental protection can we afford and how should we use our limited resources? Or: what is the tightest limit we can realistically set, which is compatible with the scoring results?

Less formal versions of this procedure can be found in "substitution analysis" for pollution prevention measures in the workplace: the toxicity profile of a substance in use is compared with the profile of a promising substitute. Only if there is a wide variation between the two will the substitute be adopted [3].

In the MOE system, certain decisions have to be made. For example, we need a decision procedure when there are no data for any given end-point. One option is to score 10, the maximum, on precautionary grounds, or on the contention that substances ought to have been tested for the end-point, prior to being put on the market. Uncertainties and non-scientific procedures there certainly are. But then there are uncertainties and scientifically arbitrary assumptions in risk assessment, too. In risk assessment, we can adopt models and work on assumptions

Table 1. MOE Scoring System Summary Chart

ELEMENT NAME	ENDPOINT & UNITS	0	SCORING CRITERIA 4	7	10
Environmental Transport	Percent partitioning, measured or predicted	Any single medium contains > 95% of the total amount released	No one medium contains > 95%, and only one medium contains ≥ 5% of the total amount released	Two media each contain ≥ 5% of the total amount released	Three or more media each contain ≥ 5% of the total amount released or Substance is inorganic or is adsorbed to particles < 10 um in diameter when released
Environmental Persistence	$t_{1/2}$ (days)	≤ 10	< 10 to 50	< 50 to 100	> 100
Bio-accumulation	BCF Log k_{ow}	≤ 20 ≤ 2.0	> 20 to 500 < 2.0 to 4.0	> 500 to 15000 > 4.0 to 6.0	> 15000 > 6.0

ELEMENT NAME	ENDPOINT & UNITS	0	2	4	6	8	10
Acute Lethality	oral LD_{50} mg/kg	> 5000	> 500-5000	> 50-500	> 5-50	> 0.5-5	≤ 0.5
	dermal LD_{50} mg/kg	> 5000	> 500-5000	> 50-500	> 5-50	> 0.5-5	≤ 0.5
	inhal. LD_{50} mg/m³	> 15000	> 1500-15000	> 150-1500	> 15-150	> 1.5-15	≤ 1.5
	aquatic LC_{50} mg/L	> 1000	> 100-1000	> 10-100	> 1-10	> 0.1-1	≤ 0.1
Sublethal Effects, Non-Mammals	aquatic						
	EC_{50} mg/L	≥ 20	2-< 20	0.2-< 2	0.02-< 0.2	< 0.02*	< 0.02*
	MATC, mg/L	≥ 2	0.2-< 2	0.02-< 2	0.002-< 0.02	< 0.002*	< 0.002*
	NOAEC, mg/L	≥ 0.2	0.02-< 0.2	0.002-< 0.02	0.0002-< 0.002	< 0.0002*	< 0.0002*
	terrestrial						
	subchronic NOEL, mg/kg/d	≥ 1000	100-< 1000	10-< 100	1-< 10	< 1*	< 1*
	chronic NOEL mg/kg/d	≥ 500	50-< 500	5-< 50	0.5-< 5	< 0.5*	< 0.5*
						*in one genus	*in different genera

Sublethal Effects, Plants						
Water, mg/L; Air, mg/m³; Soil, mg/kg						
% Growth Reduction:						
≤ 5 (= NOAEL) water	> 10	> 1-10	> 0.1-1	> 0.01-0.1	0.001-0.01	< 0.001
air	> 100	> 10-100	> 1-10	> 0.1-1	0.01-0.1	< 0.01
soil	> 100	> 10-100	> 1-10	> 0.1-1	0.01-0.1	< 0.01
> 5-50 (=EC₅₀) water	> 100	> 10-100	> 1-10	> 0.1-1	0.01-0.1	< 0.01
air	>1000	> 100-1000	> 1-10	> 1-10	0.1-1	< 0.1
soil	>1000	> 100-1000	> 10-100	> 1-10	0.1-1	< 0.1
> 50 water	> 1000	> 100-1000	> 10-100	> 1-10	0.1-1	< 0.1
air	> 10000	>1000-10000	> 100-1000	> 10-100	1-10	< 1
soil	> 10000	>1000-10000	> 100-1000	> 10-100	1-10	< 1
Sublethal Effects, Mammals* oral NOEL mg/kg/day	> 1000	> 100-1000	> 10-100	> 1-10	> 0.1-1	≤ 0.1
inhal. NOEL mg/m³	> 3000	> 300-3000	> 30-300	> 3-30	> 0.3-3	≤ 0.3
Terratogenicity mg/kg/day	no terata, or terata only at > 1000	terata or developmental anomalies at > 50-1000	terata or developmental anomalies at > 10-50	terata or developmental anomalies at > 1-10	terata at > 0.1-1, without overt maternal toxicity	terata at ≤ 0.1 without overt maternal toxicity
Genotoxicity/ Mutagenicity in vivo and in vitro cell assays	not genotoxic or mutagenic, negative results in vivo and in vitro	mutagenic in in vitro assays only; negative in vivo	mutagenic in prokaryotic cells only; negative results in eukaryotic cell assays	causes DNA induction or repair, with no direct interaction with nuclear material	causes clastogenic effects, sister chromatid exchange, crosslinks; no evidence of mutation	mutagenic in vivo (no negative results from in vivo assays)
Carcinogenicity human and animal bioassay data	no tumors in adequate studies on at least two species, and does not interact with genetic material	tumors in only one animal species, negative results in others	causes benign tumors in more than one species, and does not interact with genetic material; promotor only; or causes cell transformation in vitro only (negative evidence in vivo)	tumorigenic in bioassays at doses causing metabolic enzyme saturation, or associated with lesions that predispose to tumors. No interaction with genetic material.	indirect-acting carcinogen, no interaction with genetic material	direct-acting carcinogen that interacts with genetic material

*The Sublethal Effects, Mammals criteria are based on studies of ≥ 90 days duration. If only shorter-term subchronic studies are available, the data are modified as follows, for scoring purposes: Study duration 28-89 days – divide result by 10; Study duration ≤ 28 days – divide result by 100.

which maximize or which minimize risk [4]. Both are equally legitimate from a scientific point of view: it depends on whether policymakers want to pursue a precautionary approach or whether they want to disturb chemical use patterns as little as possible. No scientific evaluation is value-free.

WHY SHOULD POLICYMAKERS CONSULT THE EXPERTS?

In the debate so far, there is no need for policymakers to rely on expertise outside the government. There are usually in-house resources enough to draft hazard assessment procedures and risk assessment protocols. But policymakers will usually want advice from sources outside the government, e.g., at the committee stage of legislation. Among the sources will be scientific experts. One way of soliciting advice is simply to advertise hearings and ask the public to contribute. The committee accepts written submissions from all parties, then selects a limited number to testify, on the basis of whose contribution would be the most valuable, in the short time available. This is the way things are done in Canada [5]. Scientific experts are always included in environmental health deliberations, though rarely as the central or most numerous party.

One problem is that unless the experts are well-known to the public, it is difficult to identify experts whose contribution is likely to be highly valuable. If scientists always came under a banner like the Union of Concerned Scientists or Scientists Against Health Regulation Without Our Blessing, the committee would at least know the direction of the advice it would likely receive. The committee would know in advance that its proposals were either regarded as too little or far too much, always excessive. But this situation is relatively rare. Most of the time, there is a need to evaluate or grade experts as to their usefulness. Such an evaluation is provided by S. Robert Lichter and Stanley Hoffman in *Environmental Cancer—A Political Disease?* [4], hereafter referred to as L&R with page numbers in square brackets, thus [L&R, l].

Their starting point is completely the opposite from the drift of this debate to date. L&R start from the implicit presumption—it is not asserted or argued—that for every area of health policy, there is an appropriate scientific discipline. Each discipline forms a natural constituency whose exclusive prerogative is to determine policy of which their discipline is the foundation. Policy must be based on science. Thus, "the unchallenged position of scientists as masters of their own political house has largely unraveled in the new political system in Washington" [L&R, 91]. The "relevant experts are largely ignored . . ." [in the policy process; L&R 101]. "We argue for the prudence of relying upon the consensus of the scientific community (as to the facts of the case, but not as to public values) in making policy decisions" [L&R, xii].

On the contrary, throughout the book, there is no argument as to why it is prudent for policymakers to rely on scientific experts, why scientists should be consulted at all. There is much discussion of the views of environmental activists versus those of scientists and how these parties are portrayed in the media. But the prudence of relying on experts is not argued; it is assumed. There is nothing in L&R in the spirit of the great Leibnitz: calculemus—let us reason together. There is no discussion either of the relationship between science and policy: the "public values" are to be those of scientists since they are the natural constituency to consult over policy issues.

That scientists as the proper arbiters of policy should be presumed without debate comes from the splendid mutant notion of "science policy" [L&R, 91], a blatant conflation of distinct concepts that was demolished by Barry Commoner in a work, predictably, not referenced in L&R [6]. Policy is about values while science is about facts and theories.

One central question addressed by L&R is to identify and describe "an expert consensus on cancer causation" [L&R, 101]. It will then be axiomatic that this consensus will provide the rationale for public health measures aimed at the causes of cancer and thus their consequences in society. A policymaker who goes against the scientific consensus will realize measures that are ill-founded and, therefore, futile, ineffectual, or socially disruptive and counter-productive.

L&R go about their project by sponsoring a survey of experts (1993). They polled 401 experts, randomly selected from the American Association for Cancer Research (AACR), who listed either carcinogenesis or epidemiology as their field of specialization. The aim was to determine expert opinion on the science of cancer causation. The experts were mainly academics who had published extensively in peer-reviewed journals; 92% said on the phone that they were currently involved in research on the causes or prevention of cancer [L&R, 102-103].

On the face of it, selecting epidemiologists and carcinogeneticists as the relevant experts for the survey was a sound idea, since these are likely to have the most relevant opinions on cancer causation. But when this move is explored, it is less convincing than it seems. Many of the controversies in epidemiology occur when a potential hazard is newly recognized, such as electromagnetic radiations and their effects on office workers, linemen, and on children living near high-voltage electrical sources. The experts doing the research notice a connection between apparent effects and potential causes and a controversy erupts [7]. Controversy is occasionally a dispute about statistical significance. More often, the lines are drawn between those who are convinced that "there is something there" and those who aren't. The controversy then centers on the methodology of the studies. Since there is no such thing as the perfect epidemiological study, any study can be faulted on methodological grounds and used as the occasion for discrediting apparently positive results. Since most epidemiologists do not in fact study health physics, most will express the view that as a potential cause of cancer, electromagnetic radiations are dubious or a minor cause in the big picture.

All this can be quite bewildering to the educated layperson who has to evaluate the controversy in relation to public policy. Epidemiologists are a quarrelsome bunch. We can see this in the controversy over the pesticide Alar [L&R, Table 4.2, 107]. Most experts rated Alar low as a possible cause of cancer and as a minor concern. But, of course, the effects of Alar are less certain than tobacco smoke and of course the risks to the public are smaller in size than tobacco. This is on L&R's assumption that risk analyses are the only scientific grounds for policy [L&R, x, 33, 36 ff, 39, 82]. L&R imply that Alar should not be taken seriously because, unlike activists and journalists [L&R, Figure 5.5, 161], scientists rate it of low concern. This is like saying that while a big war is going on, no one should be concerned about little wars. But Alar is easy to fix: you just ban the pesticide, with the important proviso that it not be replaced by something just as bad [L&R, 77] [8]. If the experts then reply that the costs outweigh the benefits [L&R, back cover, quoting Bruce N. Ames], the response must be that the experts are no more experts on cost-benefit accounting than you or I or the Man in the Moon.

It gets worse. Reputable epidemiologists differ greatly as to the relationship between statistical associations and inferences of causality, with studies establishing a tenuous relationship between hazards and their supposed effects subject to skepticism as to whether they indicate anything at all about causality [9]. Epidemiologists who believe that such studies do not indicate a causal connection would disqualify themselves as informed commentators over most of those hazards that have attracted public controversy in recent years. The extreme case is to deny that epidemiology establishes causation at all, a position that is nonetheless philosophically defensible.

As with epidemiology, so with carcinogenesis. We should not expect an expert on metastasis to have an informed opinion on the causes of cancer. An expert who studies the mechanism whereby asbestos fibers in the lungs lead to cancerous tumors may not have an informed opinion on the relationship between the number of fibers inhaled to the incidence of lung cancer, estimates of which form the basis for workplace exposure limits. An expert on mutagenesis, such as Bruce N. Ames, may not be an expert on carcinogenesis [10]. Experts who say they work in the area of cancer prevention may confine their work to early detection and intervention (secondary prevention). If so, they are not experts on primary prevention, i.e., on how to prevent outbreaks of cancer in the first place.

When the L&R survey addresses particular policy issues, it is even more suspect. When asked whether the United States faced a cancer epidemic, 67% of experts said No and 31% said Yes [L&R, Figure 4.1, 110]. Since an epidemic can consist of a handful of cases, the correct answer would have to be affirmative. The question is too vague to be useful. Besides, an expert on the epidemiology or carcinogenesis of radon may have nothing valuable to say about the patterns and the incidence of cancer generally.

Another question in the survey was "Should chemicals and additives be banned from food and drugs if they ever cause cancer in any species ?" To this question, 85% of the respondents said No. But this question is a straight policy question, the expert answer to which is no more or less pertinent than that of the educated lay person, in fact less so if it claimed that expertise in something or other gives their opinions special weight. Policymakers can choose any one of a number of criteria for policy. "Carcinogen" can be defined in a number of ways, including evidence from structure-activity relationships, which now play a central part in chemical evaluation by the U.S. federal government. Other governments use different criteria. Neither can be said to be scientifically right or wrong: the choice will depend on what policies you want to pursue and on how to make the best use of evaluation resources.

Again, the question: "Are cancer-causing agents unsafe regardless of the dose?" If this is a factual question, the 9% who said Don't Know gave the correct answer. For the vast majority of carcinogens, it is simply not known whether there is a threshold of harm. We cannot even construct a well-founded dose-response curve, never mind establishing a threshold of safety [11]. When we look at the way that thresholds are actually used in the construction of policy, they appear not as statements of fact but as assumptions as to where we should draw the line over permitted exposures. They are rules of procedure, not facts. For instance, most health physicists work on the assumption that there is no lower threshold of harm from exposure to ionizing radiations. It is idle to ask whether it is true or false that there is a threshold.

Further, "Should human cancer risks be assessed by giving animals the maximum tolerable dose of a suspected cancer-causing agent?" A reasonable answer is No (63%), but this does not tell us what "tolerable" means in scientific practice, nor is it evident that this bears any relation to the reality of the laboratory. If we did a 90-day animal test for chronic toxicity at the "maximum tolerable dose," we would expect all or most of the surviving test animals to die shortly after the ninetieth day. That things are not done this way, can be verified by consulting the authoritative Organization for Economic Co-operation and Development (OECD) Guidelines on Chemical Testing: "The highest dose level should be sufficiently high to elicit signs of minimal toxicity without substantially altering the normal life span due to effects other than tumors" [12].

Later, L&R state [Figure 5.3, 154] that 27% of experts polled, rejected the idea that we can base human cancer risks on animal tests; this is supposedly "based on" the AACR survey. But this is a supposition completely different from the question of tolerable doses given to test animals. By an amazing coincidence, the 27% of respondents who said that test animals should not be given the maximum tolerable dose is the same figure for those who (we are told) rejected the idea of basing human cancer risks on animal studies. The International Agency for Research on Cancer, a prestigious public body, does indeed classify carcinogens on the basis of animal test evidence, as do most other cancer experts [13]. But policymakers do not have to infer human cancer risks from animal evidence. They can simply accord a lower degree of regulatory oversight to animal carcinogens than they do to known human carcinogens. The controversies over extrapolation of animal evidence to human cancer risks, [L&R, 256], then become irrelevant. L&R are forced to address the issue of extrapolation of animal test evidence to humans because of their axiom that the regulation of environmental health hazards must always be risk-based.

L&R are at their worst when they deal with scientists' ratings of levels of confidence in expertise on environmental cancer [L&R, Table 5.2, 162]. "Expertise on environmental cancer" can mean a whole range of different things. Bruce Ames is at the top of the list but (from his articles cited) he knows nothing worth knowing about cancer epidemiology. If we wanted to know about the cancer epidemic in industrialized societies, we should certainly solicit the opinions of Richard Doll, Richard Peto, and John Higginson. But we would not go to the late Irving Selikoff, who was an expert in asbestos-related cancers. Experts may have 100% confidence in Selikoff's opinions on asbestos and cancer, but none at all when it comes to his views, if he ever had any, on the relationship between diet and cancer. Similarly, scientists may have a high regard for Samuel Epstein's peer-reviewed articles but no confidence in his views on cancer policy. What we have here is a full-blooded blend of asking for subjective opinions about the wrong objects of scientific inquiry, a case of ad hominem and ignoratio elenchi in a single Fallacy of the Grand Slam. This is an intellectual accomplishment unique in the annals of the cancer wars. Science reduced to a popularity contest. A little course in Logic 101 would not go amiss. After all, L&R are professors of media and political science. We should not expect them to be experts in logical thinking.

Why then should policy-makers consult the experts at all? After all, we do not expect a gifted carpenter to be an expert on housing policy. Nor are ace fighter pilots experts on air power. Where this has proved to be the case, as with Adolf Galland and Chuck Yaeger, it is arguably because they had experience of high command before they became civilian experts on policy, not because they had been brilliant fighter pilots with a well-deserved public reputation.

The answer to the question about experts is a simple one: experts are to be consulted whenever policymakers consider their advice to be essential or useful.

Like carpenters and fighter pilots, scientific experts are capable of saying some exceedingly stupid things. Sir Richard Doll has contended that the children of Sellafield nuclear workers in the United Kingdom contracted leukemia because their over-clean homes made them susceptible to leukemia viruses.

He goes on. Since most cancers are caused by naturally occurring substances, the best thing to do is research on strategies whereby human systems can counter the action of these natural carcinogens (Doll and Ames). The body has natural defense mechanisms against synthetic chemicals, such as DNA repair, but evidently none against natural carcinogens which are allegedly thousands of times more important. That is why we need to redirect research. This is the sort of stuff we would expect from an imaginative high school student, not two of the world's most distinguished scientists.

A CASE STUDY:
OCCUPATIONAL HAZARDS [L&R, 68-72]

L&R begin by stating that the figures for cancers caused by work have been variously estimated as 6% of the total (Higginson & Muir) for men, 2% for women (Wynder and Gori) and 4% (Doll and Peto), with a lower limit of probability at 2% and a higher limit of 8%. Then came a federal government study in 1978, estimating that between 20% and 38% of cancers were occupational. "Long-simmering conflicts with management over workplace safety made labor leaders ready believers once the OSHA paper estimates were published" [L&R, 72]. As an historical perspective, this is dubious. Chronic diseases of work have been a concern of labor for centuries. The latest round of concern arose in the 1960s with the publication of *Work Can Be Dangerous to Your Health* in 1972 and *The Hazards of Work—How to Fight Them* in 1973. *Chemicals, Work and Cancer* appeared in 1980 [14]. This book downplayed the importance of epidemiology in constructing an occupational cancer policy and made only a passing reference to the OSHA paper as evidence of the seriousness of the workplace cancer epidemic.

In L&R's cosmos, labor leaders are a crowd of well-meaning duffers, always liable to be "hoodwinked" by the likes of Ralph Nader and "ready believers" when a major government study shows they had a problem on their hands which was bigger than they had ever imagined. The reality is that the labor movement employs its own experts, including risk analysts, epidemiologists, physicians, and industrial hygienists, who are quite capable of evaluating studies such as the OSHA paper on its merits, giving corresponding policy advice to the leadership.

This historical image is not unique to L&Rs' treatment of occupational hazards. We repeatedly get the impression of scientists hammering on the doors of government to persuade policymakers that their grounds for policymaking are false [L&R, 58; 94; 96 and n. 48 of Chapter 3; 113; 121]. The reality was that chemical manufacturers found a way of legitimizing their carcinogenic products through the scientific procedure of risk assessment and the adoption of thresholds in the form of "negligible risk" and "reasonable certainty of no harm" [L&R, 39].

The story of occupational carcinogenesis did not end there. The American Industrial Health Council (AHIC), an employers' group, hired Professor R. Stallones of the University of Texas to reevaluate the OSHA estimates. Stallones concluded that work-related cancers were of the order of 20%, at the lowest end of the OSHA figures, describing them as a "public health catastrophe" [15]. Thus OSHA had not "exaggerated" the figures, nor was it guilty of a "confidence trick" [L&R, 71]; it had maximized them for policy purposes. Later Canadian studies put the occupational figure at 9%, well above the high end of the Doll and Peto estimates and more than double the mean [16]. None of these developments is mentioned by L&R, though they are central to the occupational cancer controversy.

This one-sided view of the science pervades L&R's work: carcinogenic pesticides passed over lightly in favor of a past controversy over DDT [L&R, 15; 39]; the dismissal of pollution prevention as an environmental protection strategy [L&R, 37]; the failure to discuss the European middle way between socialist and capitalist approaches to environmental protection [L&R, 31-32]; downplaying the current asbestos-related cancer epidemic [L&R, 71; 180]; the supposition that nitrites are the only way to cure meat products [L&R, 77]; ignoring the evidence that trihalomethanes in drinking water cause cancer [L&R, 79 and 92]; the supposition that the only way to sterilize drinking water is by chlorination [L&R, 79 and 92]; and failing to cite sources that connect the medical administration of natural and synthetic hormones with cancer [L&R, 73-74].

The worst example is over the connection of dietary fats with cancer [L&R, 64] when in a space of two paragraphs, L&R move from saying that if certain scientific hypotheses were correct, fat would have to be regarded as a carcinogen—from this to the categorical statement that a low fat, high fiber diet will prevent up to 35% of all cancers. No mention is made of contrary theories, such as those concerning circumpolar societies, where we should expect those with a meat and fish diet, high in uncontaminated fats, to show high rates of cancer of the alimentary canal. All this is due to an obsessive desire to minimize the role of man-made chemicals in cancer causation, a truly scientific attitude.

Environmental Cancer—A Political Disease? contains many interesting observations and insights, particularly over the ideology of the environmental movement (there is no corresponding examination of the ideology of scientists). But on the rational interplay of science and policy, the book is worthless and intellectually dishonest. The book is shot through with the supposition that laypeople are incapable of evaluating the work of the experts. Judges [17] and juries routinely have to evaluate the testimony of experts. They cannot solve the problem by appealing from one expert to another. But if judges have to do this, as sure as hell, policymakers can do the same. And so must we all if we are to avoid what George Bernard Shaw referred to as the conspiracy of every profession against the laity. Experts may not be the trained dogs in Einstein's critique but their value to society will be minimal if they present themselves as a mysterious elite, beyond the pale of the grand jury of society writ large. L&R comprise a modern example of "Aristotle hath said it," whereby all criticism is to be silenced by appeal to the authority of the master. Ames and Doll take the place of Aristotle, with lay commentators such as L&R assuring us that whatever they say is true and wise. Give us a break.

REFERENCES

1. The Ontario Ministry of the Environment Scoring System for Assessing Environmental Contaminants, Queen's Printer for Ontario, 1990, page 29.
2. Opus supra, Preamble, page ii.
3. For substitution analysis, see Rossi, M., Ellenbecker, M., and Geiser, K., "Techniques in Toxics Use Reduction," *New Solutions, 2*:2, Fall 1991. For a primitive attempt to construct a rating system for chemical pesticides, see Bennett, D., "Pesticide Reduction, A Case Study from Canada," *New Solutions*, Fall 1991, pp. 59-63. Hazard Assessment is a small but well-established scientific discipline in North America (though not, curiously, in Europe). See for instance, "Criteria to Identify Chemical Candidates for Sunsetting," by Foran, Jeffrey A. Ph.D., and Glenn, Barbara A., MPH; *New Solutions*, 4:3, Spring 1994; "Comparative Evaluation of Chemical Ranking and Scoring Methodologies," CCPTC, University of Tennessee, 1994.
4. *Environmental Cancer—A Political Disease?* by Lichter, S. Robert and Rothman, Stanley, Yale University Press, 1999, p. 81.
5. The Chair of the House of Commons Standing Committee on Environment and Sustainable Development, the Hon. Charles Caccia MP, has a healthy skepticism about the testimony of all witnesses, whether they are experts, activists, or businesspeople. This has forced organizations like the Canadian Labour Congress to be utterly rigorous in their arguments and proposals, which is surely the way that public debate ought to be conducted.
6. Commoner, Barry, *Making Peace With the Planet*, Pantheon, New York, 1990, pp. 76-78. "The environmental failure has been very costly, not only in money but in burdening the still unresolved environmental crisis with a heavy heritage of poor public policy disguised as science and poor science disguised as policy" (Commoner, p. 78).
7. See for example, Carstensen, Edwin L., *Biological Effects of Transmission Line Fields*, Elsevier, New York 1987; Health and Well-Being at VDU Work, National Institute of Occupational Health, Solna, Sweden 1992; New Evidence of Cancer from Electromagnetic Fields, NIOH, Solna, Sweden 1992; "Intermittent 50 Hz Magnetic Field and Skin Tumour Promotion in SENCAR Mice, *Carcinogenesis, 15,* 1994; plus the works listed in Note 9 below.
8. Substitutions are likely to be counter-productive unless they are done in the context of an overall materials policy. See Geiser, K., *Materials Matter, Towards a Sustainable Materials Policy*, MIT Press, Cambridge, 2001, Ch 8, "Reconsidering Materials Policies," 8.4 "Detoxification."
9. For aspects of this controversy, see for instance, Rothman, Kenneth J. (ed.), *Causal Inference*, Epidemiology Resources Inc., Chestnut Hill, Massachusetts, 1988; Lillienfeld, Abraham E. M.D., M.P.H., D.Sc, and Lillienfeld, David E., A.B., M.S. Eng., *Foundations of Epidemiology* (2nd. Ed.). O.U.P., New York 1980; Hernberg, Sven, M.D., "Epidemiology in Occupational Health" *in Developments in Occupational Medicine*, Zenz, Carl M.D., D.Sc. (ed.), Chicago-London, 1980, Ch. 1; Doll R., "Interpretation of Negative Epidemiological Evidence of Carcinogenicity," IARC Scientific Publications #65, Lyon, 1985, p. 6. For the view that epidemiology does not establish causation at all, see the letter in the *New York Times* by Perl, Daniel, M.D., February 11, 1991.

10. The reason that L&R [Ch. 3, What Is Environmental Cancer?] allow mutagenesis to slide into carcinogenesis is based on (i) the contention that most mutagens are cancer initiators and (ii) the presumption that the only test for mutagenicity is the Ames test. Neither is correct. Not all chemicals with mutagenic potential are cancer initiators, far from it. There are more than a dozen lab tests in genetic toxicology. Researchers typically select a battery of such tests and can use the results for a number of purposes, e.g., a regulatory requirement that a certain set of results will indicate further testing; or to determine the future direction of research e.g., in pharmacology; or to rule out some substances from further exploration in finding practical applications for the substance or product. In these ventures, it is not as if a test or any set of tests establish whether or not a particular substance is to be classified as a "mutagen." It is rather that "mutagenic potential" is measured in relation to an objective, such as one or more of those mentioned above. The formula "mutagen, therefore cancer initiator" is misleading and simplistic.

11. Roach, S. A., and Rappaport, S. M., "But They Are Not Thresholds: A Critical Analysis of the Documentation of Threshold Limit Values," *American Journal of Industrial Medicine, 17* (1990), 727-753.

12. OECD Guidelines for the Testing of Chemicals, Paris 1993, updated regularly, Section 453, Combined Chronic Toxicity/Carcinogenicity Studies, Test Conditions—Dose Levels.

13. IARC Monographs on the Evaluation of Carcinogenic Risks to Humans, Vols. 1-69, IARC, Lyon, France, 1972-95.

14. Stellman, J. M., PhD and Daum, S. M., M.D., *Work is Dangerous to Your Health*, Vintage, New York, 1971; Kinnersly, P., *The Hazards of Work: How to Fight Them*, Pluto Press, London, 1973; LeServe, A. PhD, Vose, C. Ph.D, Wigley, C. Ph.D, and Bennett, D. PhD., *Chemicals, Work and Cancer*, Nelson, London, 1980, pp. 32-36.

15. Miller, A. B., "Planning Cancer Control Strategies," *Chronic Diseases in Canada, 13,* (No. 1 Supplement, January-February 1992); Aronson, K. J. et al., "Surveillance of Potential Associations Between Occupations and Causes of Death in Canada, 1965-1991, *Occupational and Environmental Medicine, 56* (1995), 265-269.

16. Cited in Proctor, R. N., *Cancer Wars*, Basic Books, New York, 1995, p. 67; and quoted in Firth, M., Brophy, J., and Keith, M., *Workplace Roulette, Gambling With Cancer, Between the Lines*, Toronto, 1997, p. 12.

17. Famously, Breyer S., *Breaking the Vicious Circle, Towards Effective Risk Regulation*, Harvard University Press, Cambridge, 1993.

Books About Cancer: Pragmatic Purpose,
Profound Analysis: Reviews

CHAPTER 8

The Politics of Cancer Revisited,
by Samuel S. Epstein, M.D.,
East Ridge Press, New York,
1998, 770 pages

I. THE POLITICS OF CANCER REVISITED, IN OUTLINE

The Politics of Cancer Revisited (PCR) is an update of Samuel Epstein's *The Politics of Cancer* (PC, 1978), which is included as Part I of PCR.

The PC is a 20th-century classic. It made out a convincing case that the predominant causes of cancer are environmental carcinogens in the workplace, food, consumer products, drugs, and the general environment, for example, as pollutants. While exposures to carcinogens are essentially involuntary, they are also avoidable in that it is possible or feasible to eliminate them from the human environment without significant loss of the quality of life.

The PC opened with the modes by which we demonstrate the environmental causes of cancer, took us through a wealth of case studies from the workplace, on consumer products and in the general environment, then concluded with a critique of the work of the institutions, primarily the U.S. government, the National Cancer Institute (NCI), and the American Cancer Society (ACS). Despite the billions of dollars being spent on the war against cancer, it is in fact being lost, with cancer rates soaring and neither a decline in the epidemic nor a cure for cancer in sight.

The PC appeared when U.S. cancer policy was at a crossroads. The principal government agencies [the Environmental Protection Agency (EPA), Food and Drug Administration (FDA), and Occupational Safety and Health Administration (OSHA)] had built up an anti-cancer regime which, by explicit comparison with

Great Britain [PCR, Chapter 15] was at least going in the right direction. There were signs that the leadership of the agencies would reinvigorate the battle against environmental carcinogens and carry it further. On the other hand, the federal administration embarked on a new program of deregulation and fiscal conservatism, which would have a pernicious effect on the very policies that the agencies were trying to promote. The federal initiative would result in two weapons against chemical regulation: cost-benefit analysis and risk assessment, the latter so new that Epstein, in 1978, could only describe the technique in passing and state that it was "premature."

The PCR is a rather different book. There are a number of updates (1987, 1993, and 1998) but there is no systematic attempt to bring the 1978 case studies up to date. It is disappointing, for instance, that the marginalization of OSHA under business and political pressure, is not documented. The critique of the anti-cancer agencies (NCI and ACS) is, however, utterly devastating. These agencies devote almost no resources to cancer prevention, only treatments, with the result that the war on cancer is stillborn.

The bulk of PCR is a compendium of different perspectives on environmental cancer, including lengthy statements from Epstein's allies and opponents. There are no further case studies, though there is more valuable critical study of selected medical drugs, food residues, and consumer products. There is, too, extended discussion of the cancer epidemic among women. Epstein also details the public campaigns against cancer, building on PC, which dealt mainly with the limited potential of individual and lifestyle responses. Federal regulation of carcinogens has stagnated and receded, with only the progressive actions of some individual states [notably California, New York, New Jersey, and Massachusetts] stemming the gross proliferation of known environmental carcinogens.

The PCR is multi-dimensional and it has the pragmatic political purpose of publicizing the war against carcinogens. But it is also a profound political analysis of the ideology and science of cancer, and the rationale for its reduction through effective regulation. The book can be seen as a contrast between the theorists of environmental cancer and those—mainly the chemical manufacturers and their academic and political allies—who want to give their products a clean bill of health.

II. THE THEORY OF ENVIRONMENTAL CANCER

There are four basic axioms of cancer causation: (i) the main cause of cancer is the exposure to physical and chemical agents in the environment; (ii) the greater the exposure, the greater the chance of developing cancer; (iii) cancer has a variety of conditioning factors as well as specific causes; and (iv) there is no known method of determining a limit or threshold, below which exposure to a carcinogen is "safe" [PC, 1-2].

Beyond this, there are a number of other contentions which, together with the axioms, comprise the theory of environmental cancer. Among these are: (i) the induction of benign tumors is sufficient to characterize a chemical as a carcinogen; (ii) only a small percentage of chemicals are carcinogens; (iii) carcinogenesis is characterized by irreversibility and a long latency period; (iv) there is great variation in individual susceptibility to carcinogens; (v) carcinogenicity is established either by animal testing or by epidemiology; and (vi) positive animal tests are sufficient evidence for carcinogenicity [PC, 162-163].

For any one cancer, there are thus a number of probable causes and a large variety of conditioning factors, many of them uncertain. Therefore, an effective anticancer policy will have to institute precautionary measures stronger than the total of empirical evidence indicates. For instance, it is not good enough to restrict a carcinogen in food by way of a Maximum Residue Limit (MRL), partly because of the no-threshold axiom and partly because ingesting food with more than one carcinogen in it (that is, the average diet) will make nonsense of regulation by case-by-case MRLs (the multicausality axiom). And because of multi-factoriality, there is no clear and rigid distinction between lifestyle and environmental factors. The sheer proliferation of carcinogens makes it virtually impossible for an individual to dodge them all. That is why the war against cancer has to be a collective political issue, not merely a personal and individual one.

III. THE IDEOLOGY OF THE MERCHANTS OF CANCER

The progressive theory of cancer is a well-founded scientific hypothesis. It is not value-free. There is a *moral* presumption that if cancers are avoidable, they ought to be avoided. There is a *political* presumption that where elimination of a carcinogen from the environment is feasible, there should be policies to eliminate or reduce human exposures.

The theory of the "cancer establishment" is, by contrast, problematical. In one sense, the cancer establishment does indeed have a scientific theory of cancer. If we could just understand the molecular mechanism of carcinogenesis, we could then devise a magic bullet to prevent cancer from developing in the human organism. Cancer could then be reduced to one of the lesser afflictions of humankind. As to a wider preventive public health program, the cancer establishment acknowledges that a small portion of cancers are environmental (for example, PCR 400-402: 409-411), but the vast majority are genetic in origin or due to lifestyle choices. In sum, there is no need for a regulatory program to combat cancer.

In opposing the regulatory program, establishment theory dissolves away. In its place there are a series of contentions, some practical and others allegedly scientific, whereby the merchants of cancer seek to avoid effective regulation. In different contexts, these contentions are sometimes contradictory, which befits the pragmatic and non-scientific aim of avoiding regulation. The moral premise behind the doctrine (or the several doctrines) is that it is all right to corrupt the environment with carcinogens so long as the risks are acceptable and the benefits high enough. Both science and pseudoscience are invoked to show that the risks are, in every case, minimal, acceptable, or nonexistent (for example, because of a supposed threshold), while the benefits are, supposedly, obvious.

Among the contentions that the cancer establishment adopts in its strategy to avoid regulation are:

1. *pitch the standard of proof of carcinogenicity so high that it excludes not only the agent in question, but almost every known carcinogen [PC, 164];*
2. *thus, the induction of carcinogenicity must be statistically significant at all levels and at all doses [PC, 164]; or*
3. *the mechanism of carcinogenesis must be demonstrated; a statistical association is not enough [PC, 164-5]; or*
4. *unknown "augmenting factors" (X-factors) must be excluded [PC, 164-5];* in all of these, the demand on empirical science is outrageously high, or the merchants of cancer are demanding the *logically* impossible; it is *logically* impossible *to know all* of the conditioning factors in a causal mechanism
5. *simple denial, e.g., liver cancers in one species are not evidence of carcinogenicity [PC, 165];*
6. *positive results in animal tests are not sufficient [PC, 1651; rather*
7. *positive epidemiological results are OK, but there is a threshold [PC, 97]; or*
8. *positive epidemiological results are OK, except when animal tests are negative [PC, 97];*
9. *categorize carcinogens so that the agent in question escapes classification [PC, 270];* for instance, the chemical manufacturers proposed a twofold classification of carcinogens into human and animal (that is, human non-carcinogens) with, in each class, high, intermediate, and low *potency*. In other words, even the most severe epidemic can be qualified by the low potency of the carcinogen, other factors such as lifestyle being held to blame [PC, 269-70].

Further, the manufacturers contended that:

10. *no-effect levels were still to be established [PC, 270]; and*
11. *the burden of proof is to be reversed: the regulatory agency has to establish a no-effect level [PC, 270];*
12. *risks and benefits have to be established before regulations are put in place [PC, 270);* a recent study found that only six of forty-three industry-funded studies of four highly regulated chemicals were unfavorable to the substances while of 118 studies conducted by non-industry researchers, seventy-one were unfavorable [reported in *The Ecologist,* March/April 1998: cf. PC, 189].

In other words:

14. *rig the tests [PCR, 429-30]; or*

15. *assert that animal tests conducted by the manufacturer are insufficient but then state that, in the absence of epidemiological studies, there are no grounds for regulation [PC, 331]; in other words:*
16. *no evidence of hazard is evidence of no-hazard. If all else fails, rely on*
17. *crackpot reasoning in the name of science;*
    - we have to introduce potential carcinogens into the environment; otherwise, we can't collect any human evidence that will prove them to be carcinogenic [PC 42n.];
    - the children of Sellafield nuclear workers in the United Kingdom contracted leukemia because their over-clean homes made them susceptible to leukemia viruses [a gem from Sir Richard Doll, PCR, 388];
    - since most cancers are caused by naturally occurring substances, the best thing to do is research on strategies whereby human systems can counter the action of these natural carcinogens [Doll, PCR, 393-4; Professor Bruce Ames, PCR, 413-4]; and
    - the body has natural defense mechanisms against synthetic chemicals such as DNA repair, but evidently none against natural carcinogens which are allegedly thousands of times more important [Doll again, PCR, 393-4].
18. the main causes of cancer are due to lifestyles, individual hypersusceptibility [PC, 93; 109] and causes other than the usual suspects, e.g., animal fats. In other words, blame the victim [PC, 268 and passim]; and
19. parallel to these pseudo-scientific strategies are a number of PR moves, such as exaggerating the costs and the difficulties of regulation [PC, 73; 81; 94; 134-6], threatening to move out of the country [PC, 271-4], diversionary tactics [PC, 260-266], propaganda [PC, 267] and exhausting the regulatory agencies [PC, 269-7].

IV. GLOBALIZATION AND CANCER

While the cancer battles were raging in the 1990s, two events occurred that are already having a strong impact on the war against cancer. The first of these was the North American Free Trade Agreement (NAFTA), which was signed by the United States, Canada, and Mexico in]994. Progressive critics have long been aware that there was a "social agenda" in NAFTA which is much more full-blooded and pernicious than that in the original Canada-U.S. Free Trade Agreement (FTA) of 1988. The NAFTA contains legally binding procedures which the Parties (signatories) have to go through before they regulate health hazards such as carcinogens.

These rules and procedures were essentially repeated and extended in the second big event of 1994, the signing of the World Trade Agreement. The WTO Agreement also contains rules and procedures for a wide range of different types of standards, placing even more obligations on national governments than those in NAFTA. [See NAFTA Chapter 7, Agriculture, especially Section B Sanitary and Phytosanitary Measures and Part III, Technical Barriers to Trade; Chapter 9, Standards-Related Measures; Chapter 11, Investment; The WTO Agreement on the Application of Sanitary and Phytosanitary Measures; Agreement on Technical Barriers to Trade.]

The net effect of these rules and procedures is to entrench the technique of risk assessment as a precondition for the regulation of environmental health. [Risk assessment has been invoked in the Beef Hormones and Asbestos cases before the WTO.] At the same time, the free trade agreements require governments to follow international rather than national standards (where they implement any standards at all). The net effect is that it is virtually impossible for countries to advance beyond the feeble requirements yielded by risk assessment or the generally mediocre international rules. National regulations stagnate and become outdated; no country can initiate a "breakthrough" such as the Delaney Amendment prohibiting carcinogenic additives in food (1958); we are all locked into the "toxic economy"; and environmental health is thoroughly subordinated to the demands of international trade as the verdicts of all the relevant trade tribunals have shown.

These developments will inevitably have a profound impact on anti-cancer campaigns. Currently, such campaigns focus on the need for strong national regulations, aimed at eliminating carcinogens from the environment or drastically reducing human exposures. In effect, the campaigns aim at restoring and advancing the national program as it existed in the United States in the late 1970s and before it was subverted by the merchants of cancer.

The least that can be said about such campaigns is that the tactics will have to change radically to stand any chance of success. The arena in which cancer battles are being fought (inasmuch as they are being fought at all) is now thoroughly international. The chief obstacle to an effective campaign against environmental carcinogens lies in the global free trade agreements. Until these are drastically modified, there is no hope of effective national regulatory regimes—indeed, the free trade agreements were designed explicitly to make such regimes virtually impossible. Nor, without a strong basis in national laws, is there any prospect for strong international anti-cancer treaties.

The first dilemma is in recognizing that the name of the game has changed. A second one is that focusing campaigns on elusive targets such as the WTO is no easy matter, nor are anti-cancer campaigners well versed in organizing international campaigns, which are in any case much harder to mount than national ventures. The prospects for the regulation of environmental carcinogens are even bleaker than PCR indicates.

ACKNOWLEDGMENT

The point that the cancer establishment does indeed have a scientific theory of cancer was made to me by Richard W. Clapp.

How to Win the Losing Cancer War

Cancer-Gate:
How to Win the Losing Cancer War,
by Samuel Epstein,
New York: Baywood, 2005

The occasion of this article is the publication of *Cancer-Gate: How to Win the Losing Cancer War* by Samuel S. Epstein MD. Sam Epstein is the world's leading expert and advocate on cancer causation and cancer prevention. His many works include books on the carcinogenicity of pesticides, consumer products, hazardous wastes and cosmetics, as well as more specialized studies of Bovine Growth Hormone (BGH) and breast cancer. A qualified scientist, he has published some 270 articles in peer-reviewed journals. Since his advocacy work is scientifically based, it has made him much less vulnerable to dismissive critics, though it has not prevented them from trying.

On the mainstream issue of cancer prevention, Epstein has published three books, *The Politics of Cancer* (1978), *The Politics of Cancer Revisited* (1998) and the latest, *Cancer-Gate*. Of these, *The Politics of Cancer* was not only a book on environmental health for its era; it is also a powerful critique of the cancer epidemic, cancer causation, prevention strategies, and how the war on cancer is being subverted by big business, conservative governments, and corrupt science. *The Politics of Cancer* is as much a work of political science as it is of environmental health. *The Politics of Cancer Revisited* was rather disappointing; it consisted of a reissue of *The Politics of Cancer* with a number of articles by Epstein and his opponents, not a wholesale update of the themes of the earlier book and in no sense a revisit or revision of the coherent critique in *The Politics of Cancer*.

Cancer-Gate is a great improvement on the 1998 work. "The book's chapters have been organized thematically, rather than chronologically, in four parts: Cancer Policy and Politics; Hidden Carcinogens in Food; Pro-Industry Bias, Corporate Crime, and Poorly Recognized Industrial Risks of Cancer; and an Epilogue that summarizes the reasons for the losing cancer war" [*Cancer-Gate*, xiii]. In many ways, *Cancer-Gate* is a good update of the Cancer Establishment (mainly the National Cancer Institute (NCI) and the American Cancer Society (ACS)), mammography, and occupational cancer, industrial colorectal cancer in particular. One issue is completely new: Epstein's masterly critique of the European Union's REACH program, Registration, Evaluation, and Authorization of Chemicals, which took effect on June 1, 2007, including the weakening of the REACH proposals in 2003.

Cancer-Gate still has limitations. Carcinogens in food are largely confined to the hazards of rBGH and there is no systematic treatment of either carcinogenic pesticides or consumer products.

The main limitation, of which these are symptomatic, is that almost all of *Cancer-Gate* has been previously published, without significant revision, mainly in the *International Journal of Health Services*, over the last fifteen years. One result is that the book is limited by the scope, organization, content, and thrust of the articles; another is that the updating is an irregular business. For instance, the key first chapter, Losing the War Against Cancer: Who's to Blame and What to Do About It, was written essentially in 1987 and published in 1990. The revisions to the 1987 texts are only minor and there is no editorial comment to give the reader a clue as to what is still relevant. Most other chapters date from the period 1990-2003, the mid-'90s on the average. Apart from the Epilogue, the only chapter that is truly new is the one on REACH. It would perhaps have been better to have written and organized the book systematically around several themes, for example, policy, institutions, occupational and environmental carcinogens, consumer products, pesticides, cosmetics, and winning solutions, drawing on the previously published articles as necessary.

Much has changed since *The Politics of Cancer* appeared in 1978. The 1970s started with great promise with a range of federal legislation governing environmental quality, drinking water, food safety, cancer policy, chemical testing, and workplace pollution. Since then, the whole federal program has fallen into a state of virtual collapse, with cancer prevention and the regulation of carcinogens as one leading casualty. If we are to reverse the decline and counter-attack in the cancer war, we have to understand the causes of this collapse, including corporate strategies, globalization, the business "capture" of the regulatory agencies, the death of interventionism in the U.S. Congress, the anti-regulatory provisions of free trade agreements and the use of the courts to limit government activity to the near-useless strategies of risk assessment and cost-benefit analysis. Most of this is assumed rather than explained and argued in *Cancer-Gate*.

Sam Epstein's solutions are roughly fourfold:

1. Public education and vigilant activism, of which Epstein has been in the forefront;
2. Policy changes, including the policies that inform legislation, such as those governing the cancer agencies;
3. Promotion of the right to know, so we know what we are being exposed to. We have to realize the right to know in spite of what business is adept at concealing; we can evaluate the shoddiness and fraudulence (or not) of industry data and chemical testing and we can discern the rationale (such as it is) for regulatory decisions, for example, the registration, authorization, and approval or licensing of chemicals; and

4. Proper legislation to implement cancer prevention and the regulation of carcinogens.

The first three points are well covered in *Cancer-Gate*, particularly the critique of existing cancer policies and agencies (Part I) and the poverty of Industry-Derived Safety Studies (Part III, Chapter 16). The last, concerning the legislative and regulatory program, is the least well argued. Here, Epstein's recommendations are based on a reiteration of those in *The Politics of Cancer* (*Cancer-Gate*, 16-17). In the legislative program, "Congress must resolve the major inconsistencies in a wide range of laws on environmental and occupational carcinogens." One recommendation is "cradle-to-grave" legislation as the basis for regulating carcinogens (*Cancer-Gate*, 19). Epstein sees it in combination with economic instruments and incentives for prevention. It needs to be pointed out, however, that cradle-to-grave concerns chemical management, a very different thing from the agenda of prevention, which is based on eliminating carcinogens from the environment. A second strand is white-collar crime, such as the withholding, distortion, or falsification of health and environmental data (*Cancer-Gate*, 106-9). A third is the enshrinement of the right to know in law. Epstein emphasizes the importance of state and local legislation, often enough in the face of federal preemption. It is one of the down-sides of a strong federal authority over environmental health and environmental protection, something that Canada, for example, lacks: a strong federal authority is a good thing only when the federal government decides to exercise it. The updating of these proposals in the Epilogue (2005) is disappointing: it is largely confined to the overhaul of legislation governing the cancer agencies.

There are three other areas where Epstein discusses policy and its relation to legislation: the Precautionary Principle; Pollution Prevention and Toxics Use Reduction (TUR); and references to Canada.

THE PRECAUTIONARY PRINCIPLE

In endorsing the REACH program, Epstein says rightly that it rests on the Precautionary Principle, which business, on the whole, strongly opposes. The nature of this basis is, however, unclear. Many formulations of the Precautionary Principle, for example, the one in the Rio Declaration 1992, stress that action on the environment should not be contingent on full scientific certainty. This view suggests that the Precautionary Principle should be invoked only where the knowledge-base is, for any reason, incomplete. Yet, as Epstein points out, we should adopt a precautionary approach whether or not the knowledge-base is complete. An example is asbestos. Here, the knowledge-base is as complete as it needs to be: we can base policy on risk assessment, where measures will be commensurate with the calculated risk or on a precautionary approach, which bypasses risk assessment in favor of measures that eliminate all exposures, that is, a ban. There is controversy over the reactive (risk) approach versus the precautionary approach; the dilemma has been construed, wrongly, as a scientific versus a non-scientific approach. Neither approach is more or less scientific than the other: the approaches use science in different ways. The choice of one approach over the other is political, not scientific. In this, a precautionary approach is one thing; action based on the Precautionary Principle is another. The Precautionary Principle does not tell us what action to take, only that some action should be taken. That action could be risk-based or precaution-based. It is no wonder that Epstein says that, so far as REACH is concerned, the term "Prevention Principle" is more appropriate than the Precautionary Principle. The part played by the Precautionary Principle is to require the generation and publication of data: this is the "essential precaution" (*Cancer-Gate*, 155-6).

Some formulations of the Precautionary Principle, such as the Wingspread version and the proposals adopted by the Swedish Parliament in 2001 (*Cancer-Gate*, 154-5), incorporate burden-of-proof issues into the precautionary prescriptions. The burden of proof is certainly a political issue: when the public challenges decisions in court, it has to prove that the product, process, or substance is unsafe, rather than the producer having to prove safety. It is wrong. However, the connection between precaution and the burden of proof is not obvious; on the face of it, they are different things. When it is demanded that business prove something safe, it is often enough a misconstruction of how the regulatory process works—or should work. The process is that business submits the relevant information and approval is granted by the government, to the satisfaction of the regulatory agency. In some cases, the government declares a product safe, or safe enough, that is, that risks are negligible or acceptable. It is the government, not business, that determines safety; the problem is that the process is flawed, not that business does not have to prove safety. In some Canadian cases, the situation is even worse: key federal statutes, such as the Pest Control Products Act and the Food and Drugs Act do not spell out any criteria for setting a standard or authorizing a product. In the absence of any transparency about the regulatory process and the data used in decision-making, government decisions must be seen as arbitrary and permissive. Business has to go through the motions; if it does so, approval is invariably assured.

In several places in *Cancer-Gate*, Epstein suggests that the government's cancer policy should be driven by the views of independent scientists or by representatives of labor and NGOs. Occasionally, the two groups are combined, even though public advocates represent an interest while scientists are supposed to be impartial. The point remains the same: the responsibility for regulation belongs to government, however they choose to act on advice or transfer authority to a regulatory agency. Legislation and court decisions determine where the burden of proof should lie.

Some environmentalists have walked into a trap. Critics of the Precautionary Principle demand that it be operationalized, seeking some way of deriving concrete policies from the general principle. If the arguments above are well-taken, it is an impossible task, since the Principle does not tell us to do anything in particular or how to implement policies. The Principle cannot generate any particular policies; it cannot be operationalized. The best way to defend the precautionary approach is to argue that it is politically wiser and no less scientific than reactive, risk-based, approaches, which are flawed in their scientific rationale as well as ineffectual in protecting health.

POLLUTION PREVENTION AND TOXICS USE REDUCTION (TUR)

There are two distinct strategy directions in the regulation of toxic chemicals. The first is to place obligations on manufacturers, importers, and distributors of toxic chemicals. These are questions of authorization to introduce or to continue to put chemicals into the market. They involve questions of restrictions, conditions, partial or total bans, and phase-outs. The second is to place obligations on the users of chemicals, that is, those employers who use chemicals in the production of goods and services. Some schemes combine the two, for example, the original REACH proposals would have placed obligations on the "downstream users" of chemicals. In general, however, regulatory regimes adopt one type of approach rather than the other. Realistically, it is unlikely that any regulatory authority in North America would adopt a full-blooded dual approach.

Epstein repeatedly refers to the leading case of the second type of approach, the Massachusetts Toxics Use Reduction Act of 1989 (*Cancer-Gate*, 97-9; 150; 167). He also could have cited a large number of similar Acts, such as the subsequent, progressive examples of New Jersey, Oregon, and Minnesota. Epstein's treatment of TUR is, however, rather out of focus, collapsing the two types of approaches distinguished above. One way that he does this is to see the first approach (obligations placed on chemical manufacturers) as consisting of two phases: the regulation of carcinogens new to the market, with a second phase, the regulation of existing carcinogens through "reduction of toxics in use." Another way is to require "industries manufacturing or processing HVP [High Production Volume] chemicals . . . to implement toxics use reduction programs." In these ways, two types of obligation are placed on chemical manufacturers, rather than one set of obligations on manufacturers and another set on downstream users. The Massachusetts-type legislation, however, puts obligations on downstream users; the system operates irrespective of any obligations put on manufacturers. A possible source of confusion is that TUR legislation applies to chemical manufacturing plants as well as to those facilities using chemical products. It is still a very different thing from authorization of chemicals and restrictions on what chemicals can enter the market.

Where the two approaches overlap is over the question of chemical substitution: the replacement of a toxic substance by an alternative non-toxic or less toxic chemical. In the original REACH proposal, it was expected that one of the criteria for the authorization of about 1,400 highly dangerous chemicals would be the economic and technical feasibility of alternatives. But this was weakened in 2003, so that substitution is to be "encouraged" rather than required (*Cancer-Gate*, 168). With the virtual abandonment of substitution, REACH now looks much more like a notification system dealing with disclosure of information rather than an authorization system, placing restrictions on the introduction of chemicals into the market. Substitution at the chemical user level is also one of the long-standing techniques of TUR, though Epstein considers it a recent addition to the Mass. TUR Act (*Cancer-Gate*, 167). That substitution is a powerful preventive technique is evidenced by the extreme nervousness of the industry on the issue, even though their websites list it routinely as one pollution prevention technique among others.

REFERENCES IN *CANCER-GATE* TO CANADA

Epstein discusses Canadian moves toward cancer prevention at several points in *Cancer-Gate*. These include favorable references to the Canadian Breast Cancer Screening Study and unfavorable references to the Canadian asbestos industry and the limited moves toward prevention on the part of the Canadian Cancer Society (CCS). This agency has, so far, advocated a ban on the cosmetic use of pesticides and endorsed the Precautionary Principle. There is a passing reference to an important issue, which is the handling of the Precautionary Principle on the part of the Canadian government, beyond the position taken by the CCS. Epstein takes the story only up to 2001, when the government "effectively rejected this principle." There were two principal public advocacy submissions to the government under the umbrella of the Canadian Environmental Network, one by the Canadian Labour Congress and the other, which Epstein cites, by the Canadian Environmental Law Association (*Cancer-Gate*, 123). The way that the government nullified the Precautionary Principle was to subsume it under the existing policy of risk management, with its threefold components of risk reduction, risk communication, and risk assessment. Since the risk management framework is a reactive rather than a preventive one, the Precautionary Principle can do no more than act as a qualifier in a policy that is largely ineffectual in protecting environmental health.

Since then, there have been some moves toward cancer prevention in Canada. Epstein underestimates the huge contribution that the environmental movement has made in securing a large number of municipal by-laws banning or restricting the cosmetic use of pesticides, which is beginning to have an impact on American activism. This underestimation is possibly caused by the fact that Epstein favors "commanding heights" solutions over local activities.

The various provincial cancer agencies have made moves in the direction of prevention, though they focus largely on lifestyle rather than the environmental causes of cancer. There is a national body called the Canadian Strategy for Cancer Control (CSCC), under the auspices of the new Public Health Agency of Canada. A sub-committee of the CSCC on Occupational and Environmental Exposures has produced a Best Practices Report dealing with prevention strategies in the workplace, the community and on the part of employers and governments. Such moves will only be effective if they are taken up by the public, governments, and the cancer agencies.

Recently, there has been a labor-environmental proposal to introduce Toxics Use Reduction into the Canadian Environmental Protection Act (CEPA, 1999), which is up for revision. The proposal would institute pollution prevention measures only in the limited number of workplaces covered by CEPA. There are further strategies designed to implement the federal policies in the legislation of the Canadian provinces, which have powers in the area of pollution prevention comparable to those of the American states. The NGO proposal is based on the Massachusetts TUR Act, which of course covers the whole range of toxic chemicals used in workplaces, not just carcinogens. Where the Canadian proposal differs from the Massachusetts law is that the former lists carcinogens—those in the International Agency for Research on Cancer (IARC) Classes 1 and 2A—over which employers must take measures toward elimination, not just use reduction. This proposal grows out of the substitution requirement (unique in Canada) for IARC carcinogens in the province of British Columbia. The fact that the BC Workers' Compensation Board regulation is poorly enforced only underscores the need for worker and community activism.

The reality is that Canada is way behind the U.S. on cancer prevention. There are moves to set up a labor-environmental Cancer Prevention Coalition, one of the key strands being the CSCC Best Practices Report. There is already some impact of the Best Practices Report on the cancer agencies, particularly in the areas of substitution, the Precautionary Principle, and the articulation of precautionary approaches to environmental carcinogens. The basis of the national coalition will be the grass roots rather than big names and powerful voices for cancer prevention—if indeed we had any, which we don't. A start has been made by such local and regional groups as the Labour-Environmental Alliance Society of British Columbia and the Toronto Cancer Prevention Coalition. On the part of some of the leading lights, there is a good reason for building a network of local labor-community alliances. At present, the regulation of carcinogens is in a poor state. The normal routes of parliamentary lobbying and advocacy will be useless unless there is a groundswell of grass roots activity to prove that prevention is both popular and feasible—and represents a political constituency. The Canadian Labour Congress, for instance, has produced a Practical Manual for Labour-Community Cancer Prevention Campaigns, which is likely the first of its kind and a good guide as to how to set up and work a local cancer prevention campaign. It is available on the CLC website at www.clc-ctc.ca

None of this detracts from the achievement of *Cancer-Gate*. But it should be evident from this review that Epstein's principal accomplishment remains *The Politics of Cancer*. If this magnificent work were all that he wrote, it would be enough to secure his undisputed leadership in cancer prevention and the starting point for us all.

ACKNOWLEDGMENT

Thanks are due to Larry Stoffman of UFCW-Canada for his contributions to the section on Canada.

CHAPTER 9

The Secret History of the War on Cancer, by Devra Davis, Basic Books, New York, 2007: Review

Devra Davis, PhD., MPH is the Director of the Center for Environmental Oncology at the University of Pittsburgh Cancer Institute and Professor, Department of Epidemiology, Graduate School of Public Health. For Davis, there are two aspects to the question of fighting cancer: what would count as winning the war and how has the secret history impeded the battle, contributing to its failure or at least qualifying its success. As to the first, the war could be won by a huge increase in the survival rate of cancer sufferers (effective treatments and a cure) or by instituting prevention measures that would reduce the incidence of cancers in the first place—or both. Davis acknowledges that the incidence has declined and survival rates for some cancers have increased in the past generation and occasionally hints at a possible breakthrough in avoiding exposure to specified carcinogens through a study of the immune system and micro-biological techniques. But the predominant theme is the reduction of incidence through prevention measures, the radical reduction of exposures to carcinogens or the elimination of cancer-causing substances and processes from the human environment. Broadly, the chief obstacle to doing this is the withholding or concealing of information on the causes of cancer: no prevention measures are possible if the causes of different cancers are either unknown or known only to the purveyors of the carcinogens in question.

The Secret History of the War on Cancer is not a systematic book. For instance, there are no continuous threads of argument over the two themes of prevention and treatment, nor the ways in which research findings can be used as a weapon in the war on cancer. As will be argued, this lack of systematic analysis is on balance an asset rather than a criticism. The book is not centrally or essentially a work of health science but what might be called literary social history. Statements of fact, narratives and analysis are invariably colored by descriptions of social setting, the personalities of the actors and how academic and scientific issues are given a gloss through Davis's own personal attitudes and family history. Apart from an extended discussion of cervical cancer, the approach of the book is to examine a series of carcinogens and draw conclusions, either similar or contrasting, about their significance for the war on cancer. The main carcinogens examined are tobacco smoke, asbestos, coke oven emissions, toxic pollution and wastes, vinyl chloride, benzene, cell phones, CT scans, and the artificial sweetener aspartame, so that the study deals equally with work, consumer issues, and the social environment. Other topics covered are by way of anecdotes or Davis's personal experience as well as observations made in passing or to illustrate a general point, such as the discussion of cancers among researchers and medical practitioners. Yet most of these peripheral or cursory treatments are properly documented and annotated: Davis does not sacrifice scientific integrity in her work of literary social history.

Nearly all of the main carcinogens discussed have been subjected to secrecy, the withholding or concealing of information that would either magnify the seriousness of the issue or point to a precise cause and thus a culprit. The modes of this secrecy are roughly fourfold:

1. *Trade Secrecy and Proprietary Information.* This occurs when a producer or purveyor of a carcinogen has information which can or must be concealed under official government authority or legal sanction. Thus, for instance, a workplace Material Safety Data Sheet (MSDS) may have information that is officially designated a trade secret (including scientific studies that would reveal the identity of the material), meaning that workers and employers can have no access to this information, except (sometimes) under strict conditions. If the seriousness of the issue cannot be determined, we can't institute a coherent series of prevention measures in the workplace. Another example is information that is given to the government by the manufacturer or importer of a (suspected or potential) carcinogen for evaluation purposes. In such cases where the information is claimed as proprietary, the public has no way of knowing whether the resulting regulatory measures are appropriate or adequate. Even information on the health status of workers can be claimed as a trade secret by the employer.

2. *De Facto Business Confidentiality.* Big business has an aura of secrecy, in origin through the protection of competitive advantage but extending this to the concealing, as far as possible, of any and every item of information having a bearing on the touted benefits or detriments of a product, the research that informs it and information relating to production processes and the composition of products. A general rule is that an item of information or analysis that is not required to be divulged will remain secret. Often enough, the public has no knowledge of what items of information and knowledge exist within the premises of a business; we do not know the extent of our own ignorance.

3. *Control of Information and Suppression of Research Findings.* Davis's book is replete with examples of researchers, as university scientists or as independent contractors, who have been denied permission to publish their findings (except sometimes in a distorted fashion) and who have been intimidated, threatened with legal action, or fired for breaking the rules laid down by a corporate employer. As will be seen, this has implications for the independent integrity of research projects, for law reform, and academic freedom.

4. *The Availability of Information.* Davis has two prominent examples of the lack of availability of cancer studies, of which the first involves the control of information. The five-volume *History of Cancer Control in the United States, 1946-1971*, a Report to the National Cancer Institute on the Early History of the Cancer Control Program was so restricted in its circulation that Davis had to track down a xeroxed copy in the private library of Daniel Teitelbaum, a professor of toxicology in Colorado. The second example is the three-volume proceedings of the Second International Congress of Scientific and Social Campaign Against Cancer, held in Brussels in 1936. Davis describes that conference as a venue where "several centuries of cancer research flashed onto the scene, ready to coalesce into a substantial and coherent body of scientific understanding about the environmental causes of cancer." Instead, the accomplishments of the conference were forgotten: no copy was available in the United States and Davis had to request a copy from a library in Belgium. Her point is that once the veil of secrecy is lifted, we can see just how much of the science and philosophy of cancer has progressed, then been forgotten or suppressed. Concepts which we regard as modern or contemporary have a long and thwarted history: standards of proof of hazard; the techniques of identifying cancer causation; the importance of prevention measures vis-à-vis modes of treatment; the principle of substituting non-carcinogens for carcinogens, the total enclosure of carcinogenic industrial processes—these were all familiar to the cancer community in the 1930s and had to be rediscovered two generations later. She has an intriguing theory, concerning scientific and social optimism after the end of the Second World War, to explain why these progressive ideas were forgotten.

Davis has several strands of argument as to why the war on cancer is being lost: the secrecy of the war; the wrong battles with the wrong weapons and the wrong leaders; the collusion of business, governments, and academic institutions; the revolving door of cancer researchers in and out of cancer-causing industries. But a major theme of the book, which includes but is not limited to the issue of secrecy, is what she calls the manufacture of doubt—doubts about the seriousness of the issue and doubts whether measures to reduce the incidence of cancer are really needed. As with secrecy, there are a number of ways in which doubt is manufactured by the purveyors of carcinogens. These modes of manufacturing doubt are again broadly fourfold: the suppression and distortion of research results indicating hazard and risk; creating doubt on the significance of research findings; partiality—ensuring that research projects are not independent but controlled by the purveyors of carcinogens; and modes of stalling intervention and action contingent on the establishment of hazard.

1. *The suppression and distortion of research results.* This mode of creating doubt, which is also a mode of secrecy as noted above, is political rather than scientific, such as intimidating researchers, threatening their careers, dismissal, and threatening legal action to head off the publication of research findings.

2. *Creating doubt as to the significance of research findings.* Here, the motive is political, to deny the reality of hazard, but the discourse is ostensibly scientific. Some of the elements in this strategy are:

- a play on the significance of animal versus human evidence of hazard, e.g., by demanding another type of evidence when the one indicates hazard or by casting doubt on the inferences from hazards indicated in test animals to human beings; generally, creating doubt about the type of evidence needed to establish a scientific conclusion.
- in the absence of agreement or a protocol on the standard of proof of hazard, claiming that a conclusion is really a tentative hypothesis; that there are unknown or unquantified factors at work besides the designated cause; attributing harm to individual susceptibility as opposed to systematic vulnerability; demanding expensive repetition or amplification of test results, "more research"; contending that the mechanism of carcinogenesis must be known before harm is attributed to an agent; and, in the extreme case,
- conducting no research, then claiming that there is no hazard through the Fallacy of the Misplaced Quantifier: no evidence of hazard is evidence of no-hazard.

3. *Partiality.* This works by ensuring that research projects are controlled by the purveyor of the carcinogen, rather than being conducted in independent or quasi-independent institutions, such as governments, universities, research institutes, and laboratories at arms-length from the business responsible for testing the carcinogen. Independence is of course no guarantee of integrity and, wherever research is conducted, there has to be openness and transparency as to the modes of research and the results. So the question of partiality is connected with the suppression of evidence: where the research project is opaque, the identity of the researchers concealed or the modes of a study hidden, there can be no confidence that the results are bias-free or that a potential hazard has been properly evaluated.

4. *Modes of stalling on intervention and action.* Some such modes involve the evaluation or a commentary on test results; but these strategies are essentially public relations activities, such as the promotion of "safer cigarettes" or the contention that crysotile is significantly less hazardous than other forms of asbestos. In these cases, doubts about safety are lifted by assurances that there can now be business as usual.

These strategies are currently called "issue management." Previously, hazards themselves were merely "managed" rather than eliminated or reduced. Now the issue itself is managed so that it goes away, a testament to the worthlessness of most recent management text books.

THE RECEPTION OF THE SECRET HISTORY OF THE WAR ON CANCER

The reception of *The Secret History* was mixed; there were, in particular, two hostile reviews in non-specialist journals, Dr. Richard Horton in the *New* York *Review of Books* (March 6, 2008) and Dr. Ezekiel J. Emanuel, a breast oncologist, in the *New Republic* (March 27, 2008). Horton begins his review with a critique of the war on cancer and the cancer establishment similar to that of Devra Davis. A second section on the career of the epidemiologist Sir Richard Doll again partially reflects Davis's perspectives. But he then sets out an apologia for Doll's concealment of his close ties to the industries he was investigating and concludes that Davis's critique is "a partial view [that] seems unbalanced and unjust." (The only letter that the NYR printed in response was in the June 26, 2008 issue by Professor Gayle Greene, endorsing Davis's attacks on Doll's professional integrity, attacks which were by no means new in 2007.) Horton's review then degenerates into one of the most inaccurate, distorted, unfair, and misleading pieces that the NYR has ever published. Her book is a series of "loose speculations," "little more than a collection of vague exhortations to do something based on an often distorted reading of the cancer literature." One of the two big problems that Davis ought to have examined is tobacco and Davis would have done better to focus on smoking—an odd prescription since tobacco gets the most extended treatment of all in *The Secret History*!

The second big cancer problem that Horton identifies is obesity and, on this, he is joined by Dr. Emanuel, who accuses Davis of producing a hysterical and exasperating book. On the contrary, Emanuel's review is poisonous academia at its best, systematically misrepresenting Davis's views and self-righteously pursuing a double standard under the guise of scientific integrity. Here is how. Emanuel quotes the International Agency for Research on Cancer as laying down seven criteria for confirming whether or not a chemical, radiation, or some other agent causes cancer. But obesity, supposedly the main factor in a third of all cancers, would fail to meet any of the seven criteria, since we get a simple correlation, without any enquiry as to the presence of different, specified carcinogens in fat cells. The supposition that obesity itself causes cancer is mere speculation or propaganda, not science. Emanuel's contentions over obesity are not worth the paper they are written on.

One of Emanuel's accusations is that Davis advocates a series of crackpot natural remedies in treating cancer. At a glance, Davis's text, with its frequent emotional reflections and spiritual aspirations, could easily give such an impression. Davis's discussion of natural medicine, the role of lifestyle and diet in cancer prevention is, however, measured and level-headed. She emphasizes that the role of a healthy diet in cancer prevention and treatment is, and can be, a science with tangible results to date. Nor does she advocate alternative remedies alone, only in conjunction with conventional, mainline treatments. She concedes that in some cases the effectiveness of natural remedies may be a psychological matter, but this is true of some conventional treatments too.

SOME ELEMENTS OF AN ACTION PROGRAM ARISING OUT OF THE SECRET HISTORY

Communications

The prosecution of the war on cancer requires an army of footsoldiers, not merely a corps of activists and scientific advocates. We need the educated general public on our side. Books and articles are not of course, the only means of communicating campaigns to the public, nor are they now solely in the form of hard copy. But they are still a central weapon in the war. In this respect, *The Secret History of the War on Cancer* is a model because it is eminently readable and persuasive while still retaining scholarly credentials. It joins several other books in this respect, including Paul Hawken's *Natural Capitalism,* Sam Epstein's *The Politics of Cancer,* Naomi Klein's *Disaster Capitalism* and Eric Schlosser's *Fast Food Nation.* What these books have in common is that they include a focus on the part played by work and workers, both as those on the receiving end of current policies and as instruments of change.

By contrast, far too many books are dull, academic tomes, full of scholastic debate and with a dearth of prescriptions for action and change. Such scholarly debates are undeniably important in academia, but in books with a popular appeal, the results of academic debate are only useful in as much as they inform a prescription for change. Nobody should really care whether Adorno or Foucault or Marx or the author got it right in any book supposed to have a popular appeal. Such issues are the stuff of academic theses; however, a supposedly popular book that is merely a PhD thesis in between hard covers, unadapted for a general readership interested in social change, will not succeed in recruiting anyone to the progressive cause.

Academic Freedom and the Independence of Research

Traditionally, we see academic freedom as the right to express unpopular or heretical views without fear of intimidation or dismissal. And so it is, but in the area of health research, there is an additional factor: health research is a pragmatic discipline designed to influence policy, public and private, and whose results are a matter of public interest. Ideally, but in an immediate and practical sense, academic institutions and their members should conduct research which is open to public scrutiny and no projects should be accepted where there are restrictions on the public disclosure of research protocols and the results. Such is the reliance of academic institutions and researchers on corporate funding that restrictions on disclosure are the norm, not the exception. What we need is a campaign on the part of academic unions and associations to applaud research contracts where the livelihoods of the researchers are fully protected and the methods and results open to public scrutiny. This is one part of a wider issue: measures to ensure, as far as possible, that research on cancer is as independent as possible from the purveyors of carcinogens and, equally important, open to public scrutiny.

Law Reform

Just as important as removing the veil of secrecy is a theme discussed at length in *The Secret History:* the way in which the legal system sets the standard of proof of harm so high that victims of a harmful substance or process are denied legal redress. This in turn retards the progress of preventive measures and the development of less unsafe alternatives. In the Supreme Court *Daubert* case of 1993, the judges set a precedent that "the only clear evidence of human harm came from publications that analyzed statistically significant instances of human deformities or death." So the results of animal tests, a plenitude of clinical case reports, and a simple correlation of cancers with working or consumption conditions were all ruled out as evidence of harm. Conventional scientific evidence was rejected in favor of extremely expensive and inaccessible epidemiological studies. Later cases made scientific reasoning even more restrictive: the researchers, and not just the evidence, had to have the endorsement of their peers in the profession. Results from a brilliant maverick, the sort that revolutionize common practice, are ruled out. The courts, in consequence, Davis argues, should recognize more traditional and "scientifically reliable patterns of evidence." This would, in a reversal of the usual practice of science informing the law, help to recognize and institutionalize scientific standards of proof, and thus form a basis for the effective regulation of hazards. As it is, the settlement of cases out of court, however just, means that the degree of harm cannot be publicly recognized.

One of the motives behind corporate secrecy, the curtailment of research and the manufacture of doubt is to avoid legal liability for inflicting harm: what seems on the surface to be simple dishonesty is really the avoidance of legal liability. Davis has a proposal for coming to terms with past corporate wrongs: a kind of Truth and Reconciliation Commission (an idea that needs developing), whereby corporations would come totally clean in return for the lifting of liability for past harm to workers and communities. Another proposal is a comprehensive medical surveillance program for exposed workers, an idea which this reviewer does not find promising. The reason for skepticism is that medical surveillance is not essentially a preventive technique; historically, it has rarely been geared to the elimination of the causal conditions of the harm, or potential harm, that medical and biological surveillance reveals.

Health Policy in Relation to Science

Broadly, the model we adopt for dealing with health detriments is based on the accumulation of a body of scientific evidence, principally the attribution of a cause to a body-count, then measures to address the issue, commensurate with the seriousness of the detriment or the degree of certainty in establishing a cause. Devra Davis contends that this is the wrong model for health policy and she elaborates on this theme in her audio interview with the Collaborative on Health and the Environment (www.healthandenvironment.org/partnership_calls/2505) and on her own website (www.devradavis.org). The focus on preventive, pre-cautionary measures suggests that health policy should focus on the end-point (the health of individuals and communities) rather than being "science-driven"—policy as the outcome of a scientific enterprise. Thus, for example, instead of trying to determine whether and how cell phones cause cancer of the brain and auditory nerve, we *first* pursue technology to eliminate or reduce electro-magnetic field (EMF) exposure to the head of the phone user, e.g., perhaps, by earpieces. It then makes sense to undertake health studies on cell phones incorporating the best available technology, not on equipment which is really obsolescent. There is a parallel here over VDT use: the controversy over whether VDT use caused cancer and miscarriages was ended abruptly through the simple device of reducing EMF emissions by shielding and grounding the flyback transformer. More generally, preventive measures such as the substitution of non-carcinogens for carcinogens are more effective than the time and resources to prove that something really is carcinogenic. Contrary to industry propaganda, such measures are also cost-effective, reducing costs, irrespective of the health benefits, since industrial efficiency invariably increases as a result.

The Social Costs of Cancer Care

In a discussion of various techniques for the detection of breast cancer, and the resulting medical interventions, Davis says, "The marketing of mammography, ultrasound and breast MRI has a life of its own, where the opportunity to conduct hard, cold analysis is hamstrung by the fabulous profitability of the business." The implication is that no national system of medical insurance, public or private, can possibly provide a universal and equal service with such a proliferation of tests and interventions. There has to be some form of limitation on insured services, and thus of cost; otherwise we will continue to see the arbitrary and ill-informed denial of benefit and service which is characteristic of the current system of private insurance.

In all, readers will learn much that is valuable from Devra Davis's book, which is both highly informative and a pleasure to read.

PART V

From Environment to Sustainability

CHAPTER 10

Industrial Materials: A Guidebook for the Future: Review

MATERIALS MATTER—
TOWARDS A SUSTAINABLE MATERIALS POLICY,
by Kenneth Geiser, Cambridge, Massachusetts:
MIT Press. 2001, 479 pp.

Materials Matter has three objectives: to examine the history of industrial materials and the impact of their development on human health and the environment; to examine potential future routes for materials development that might be more conducive to health and environmental protection; and finally to consider what private and public policies could most effectively guide such developments [p. 15].

The first, historical, aim takes up about half of the book. It is a masterly and authoritative survey. Ken Geiser concludes that current materials policy depletes the global stocks of high-quality natural resources; dissipates those resources into the environment—as wastes or as discarded products—in forms that are irrecoverable; uses and wastes large amounts of energy in the process, pollutes the planet; converts relatively safe chemical compounds into quite toxic compounds; and exposes large numbers of people to chemical compounds that are inadequately studied [p. 198].

The basic reasons as to why all this has happened are given by Barry Commoner in his Foreword to the book. There has been little effort on anyone's part—producers, consumers and governments alike—to deliberately design materials to suit *any* system of production, let alone one dedicated to the protection of the environment and public health. Rather than developing products by a known method, enterprises develop any product that looks promising, then cast around for applications, that is, markets. As John Kenneth Galbraith so famously observed, capitalism creates human needs where none exist, both developing and supplying the means to satisfy these artificial needs. It is not as if design has failed. Rather, principles of design are based only on technical feasibility and economic desirability as construed by the producers of materials and products [p. xi].

The other half of *Materials Matter* is devoted to alternative materials policies and strategies. This account too is wide-ranging, deep and discerning, with critical analysis worthy of the giants of the field, such as Kenneth Boulding, Herman Daly, and Paul Hawken.

As to Geiser's third objective, the policies needed to guide such strategies, there are a number of intriguing and perceptive ideas put forward for discussion; but these are mainly summarized in a single, final chapter. "Strategies" here really means alternative routes to take; there is no sense of how to build a social movement to achieve the alternatives. As Geiser rightly points out, public movements have focused almost exclusively on the environmental impacts of production and their social costs, rather than industrial materials and production processes themselves. Yet the key to a sustainable materials policy lies at the heart of the system, not at its peripheries.

There are essentially three arguments, three types of rationale, advanced by the author for a sustainable materials policy, the first well-articulated and convincing, the two others less so. The first argument is from the deleterious impacts of current materials policy on health and environment; the second from the need for a sustainable future and the last from nature, the way in which the natural world works.

As to the first of these, Geiser partly summarizes and partly takes for granted the impact of current modes of industrial production on human health and ecological integrity. He then looks at current responses to these impacts which are hopelessly inappropriate and inadequate. Regulatory policy focuses on one substance at a time; studying pollutants and their impact takes up an inordinately large amount of public and private resources; and safety is addressed long after most materials have been on the market—sometimes when the substance is already obsolete [p. 14]. Establishing safe levels of exposure is a frustrating business, compromised by lack of evidence, the cost of generating information and the role of political interests of all sorts. We would all be better off finding and developing less hazardous substances [p. 336]. The ideas for alternative materials are always examined with their health and environmental consequences in mind [Part III, pp. 215-304].

At times, Geiser seems to overstate the case, for instance when he expresses skepticism over the value of chemical bans and phase-outs [pp. 350-351], rightly pointing out that substitutes can be worse than what they replace. Yet, surely, the collapse of the restriction program and its compromise by risk assessment techniques reflects as much the political climate of the United States and the power of the transnational chemical industry as it does the limitations of the project. In Europe, there is a wealth of experience and proposals to systematically ban whole classes of chemical products, such as industrial chemicals, pesticides, growth hormones, and food contaminants of all sorts. That bans need to be implemented in the context of a sustainable materials policy is Geiser's positive intervention; but that they provide a spur to innovation, there is no doubt.

The second argument, from sustainability, is based on the conventional argument that sustainable development must meet the needs of the present without compromising the ability of future generations to meet their own needs [p. 196]. Sometimes, this formula is given content and meaning by the well-known argument that we should not draw down natural capital stock and that the "resource stock should be held constant over time" [p. 203]. At other times, Geiser refers to "dwindling natural materials" as if we are depriving future generations of the resources to meet needs analogous to our own [pp. 252, 308].

But this, surely, is rather a weak argument, criticized by John Simon and others. The fact is that the earth is not running out of resources and, where a resource is threatened (such as zinc, for instance), substitutes are invariably found. This is due to market forces, which Geiser at times concedes [p. 207], stating only that they will not be enough to secure the alternative materials program. On the contrary, one problem is that current materials are too inexpensive to avoid their wasteful use and create pressure for the development of alternative materials. Proponents of the sustainability argument have wisely put the emphasis on the back end of the production process (unsustainable production and waste) rather than the front end: the impact of resource utilization on future generations. Geiser does discuss the ecological costs of resource extraction, to be remedied by keeping materials actively cycling within the economy [p. 314], but of course, this is an environmental impact argument, not an argument about draining the planet's resources. On Geiser's side, it is quite true that we are wasting resources, whether or not we are running out of them. But in view of the sub-title of the book, the sustainability argument is less important than it might appear.

The argument from nature concerns the way in which nature produces and uses materials (p. 3]. By modeling materials and their uses on the processes of nature, we would more likely fit our practices into natural, ecological systems. This is an instrumental argument; it concerns the means, rather than the ends, of the sustainable materials policy. Recycling, closed loop industrial processes and industrial ecology generally are cited as examples of this modeling of industry upon nature. It needs to be said, however, that such activities ape nature only in the most general ways. They can be justified on the basis of the argument from environmental health alone, quite apart from the general analogies with natural processes. The value of these activities is that they derive their *inspiration* from nature, which works in much more complex and interrelated cycles of "production" than general recycling systems. The actual modeling of recycling systems on nature is a less compelling argument. The main thing is to curtail the linear life cycle of current industrial processes. To the degree that this third argument is convincing, it depends on the potential success of bio-based materials [pp. 283-304], which are examined later under the heading of alternative materials strategies.

These alternative strategies are fourfold: recycling and reuse of materials; advanced and engineered materials; renewable materials and bio-based materials. The recycling and reuse of materials reduces both the volume of waste and the environmental degradation of the resource extraction process but it is seen as a strategy with limitations, partly due to the limits of physical possibility, partly because of economics, and partly because of unavoidable inefficiencies in recycling systems. This critique, though not new, is entirely valid [pp. 215-236].

Advanced and engineered materials are characterized by being created for specific purposes; they are highly processed and have a high value-to-weight ratio; they are developed and replaced with high frequency and they are often combined into new composites [pp. 240-241]. They include superalloys, structural ceramics, high-performance polymers, composites, electronic materials such as conductors, photonic materials, "smart" materials which resist extreme environmental pressures and nanoparticles with a capacity for self-assembly. Some of these products are less energy-intensive than conventional material processes, energy conservation being a sub-theme of *Materials Matter*. But few of these technologies are without serious health and environmental problems of their own, partly because they rely on conventional raw materials and partly because of the toxicity of the process, such as the production of ceramics, composites, and the silicon-based semiconductor industry. This last also uses large amounts of water and energy: cleanliness of the product does not imply cleanliness of the process. Geiser argues that technology assessment and hazard assessment should be built into the process of research and development, instead of being treated as a separate afterthought [p. 258]. It is not enough that advanced materials meet the three paramount factors of performance, efficiency, and cost.

Renewable materials are agricultural commodities used as industrial raw materials. Geiser produces a similar detailed breakdown of the sorts of commodity that could or do have industrial applications. He argues that this has benefits such as diversification of agricultural markets, the better utilization of land resources and the reduction of farm commodity surpluses. We can also take it that because of the natural origin of the materials, the toxicity of the subsequent processes is likely *in general* (though not necessarily) to be reduced. The real problem is with agricultural intensification and chemical agriculture. If these modes of agricultural production are not transformed, the environmental and health detriments of the agricultural base of renewable materials will be exacerbated, not reduced [pp. 274-281].

Bio-based materials are those produced by the transformation of natural materials or the transformation of natural materials by natural processes, albeit under artificial conditions. The examples given are biosynthesis and the bioprocessing of chemicals, for instance, through fermentation; biodegradation; biomimetics; biotechnologies such as genetically engineered enzymes, and bio-polymers. Among the advantages cited of bioprocessed materials over petro-chemical materials are: the feedstocks are typically renewable and ubiquitous; most bio-based materials are produced in aqueous environments under normal temperature and pressure; biocatalysts (usually enzymes) are highly active and selective, with few environmental detriments (unlike heavy metals); they generate energy internally and they generally produce biodegradable products and by-products [p. 302].

However, in this area, Geiser seems to understate both the opportunities and the risks. Under the heading of biomimetics, which replicates the processes of living organisms, he cites the efficiency of natural processes: for instance, the effectiveness of natural adhesives and abrasive surfaces or the toughness of natural filaments such as silk. But very few examples are given of promising experiments.

In *Biomimicry*, Janie Benyus has cited a number of instances in which researchers have gone further than identifying a natural model. They have attempted, for instance, to store energy from natural light, one route to this being to "remake nature in inorganic form," using synthetic membranes to create electrical potential. They have used the enzyme hydrogenase to produce hydrogen in the context of photosynthesis, successful for short periods of time so far. This success has been limited to date because no way has yet been found to prevent the reaction from being overcome by oxygen, which shuts down the reaction. They have used an artificially created enzyme, known as a photozyme, to manufacture vitamin C, using sunlight and photosynthesis. There have been attempts to synthesize (adapt) a gene to manufacture a silk-like protein.

Benyus also cites the first successful experiments in carbon-based computing, in which "synthesized DNA strands" are tagged with the names of variables and sorted biologically, the living equivalent of abstract computer logic realized in hardware. Since there is (arguably) no concept of waste in nature, such processes are likely to take us closer to the (impossible) ideal of Zero Waste, which Geiser examines in the context of dematerialization [pp. 317-318]. In other words, Benyus sees a potential in "green chemistry" which takes us beyond the work of Paul T. Anastasias and John C. Warner, cited later by Geiser in the discussion of detoxification [pp. 357-362], for instance, in her slogans of "no large fluxes" and "chemistry *au naturel*."

Geiser also seems to understate the risks. He observes that the possibilities of materials based on natural processes are so rich that it "appears" unnecessary to leap to gene-altering technologies in food production that raise unexplored risks. It is surely a scandal and again a testimony to unchallenged corporate power that no health and nutrition testing is required for genetically modified organisms; that the test data submitted and their evaluation by public authorities are kept secret; that tests on environmental impacts on biota and ecosystems are slight, short-term, and cursory; and that producers are allowed to ride roughshod over the public's right to know what it is eating—on the spurious grounds that such knowledge is scientifically insignificant.

Moves toward a sustainable materials policy depend on the twin concepts of dematerialization and detoxification. *Detoxification* means the reduction of the toxic characteristics of industrial materials. This could be accomplished by toxics use reduction (TUR), including substitution of less toxic substances or by changing industrial processes, so that the toxicity of materials is reduced or eliminated. *Dematerialization* means increasing the service value of products per unit of material used. This could involve recycling and reuse, designing products that use fewer materials, or substituting non-material services for material-intensive products [p. 16]. Very roughly, dematerialization reduces environmental impacts while detoxification reduces impacts on human health as well as the health of ecosystems. The two concepts are examined in as much critical detail [pp. 307-366] as the fourfold alternative materials strategies.

But here again, Geiser advances a conceptual framework through which to understand the two ideas. With detoxification, Geiser supplies a decision procedure for determining which chemicals can be considered "reasonably compatible with environmental processes," which chemicals are to be permitted to cycle between the economy and the environment and which should not. Persistence, bioaccumulation, and degradability play a part in this categorization as well as toxicity [pp. 336-340]. This decision procedure is not annotated and seems to be highly original. With dematerialization, there is a comparable schema, based on the work of Herman Daly [pp. 311-313], which in turn rests on a framework advanced by such thinkers as Barry Commoner [pp. 198-204].

Geiser is both an accomplished administrator and advocate of materials policies through his work as Co-Director of the Lowell Center for Sustainable Production at the University of Massachusetts Lowell. With *Materials Matter,* he has shown that he is a first-class historian of materials technology and a policy analyst of the most acute and discerning kind. The book more than fills a huge gap in the literature and will be used as a textbook, policy manual, and a detailed manifesto for materials policy for many years to come. *Materials Matter* is the sort of book that practitioners aspire to write as the culmination of a long career. With Geiser, all the indications are that even better things are yet to come.

CHAPTER 11

———————

'Natural Capitalism's' Bold Theory: Review

NATURAL CAPITALISM: CREATING THE NEXT INDUSTRIAL REVOLUTION,
by Paul Hawken, Amory Lovins, and L. Hunter Lovins, Little Brown, Boston, 396 pages, $26.95

In order to place *Natural Capitalism* in current social thought, we have to understand its background in environmental theory. There are roughly three types of environmental theory:

1. Theories in which ecology and nature are prime. The part to be played by human beings in natural systems is problematical, either irrelevant—in the theory known as "deep ecology"—or as a positive liability in that human activities are seen as hostile to nature. Thus, some theorists state that, in order to sustain, restore, and enhance natural systems, global human population must be reduced to a couple of hundred thousand souls. Spiritual values often inform such theories, with reverence and awe of nature giving the theory its vitality and human purpose;

2. Theories that put human beings in the world, as a part of nature—as in "social ecology—or as elements to be valued along with nature. Such theories are to varying degrees "anthropocentric"—that is, humanity displaces or complements nature in the center of the environmental stage. The two approaches converged in Rachel L. Carson's *Silent Spring* (1962), where environmental policy was seen to violate both human and natural values alike.

3. Theories in which the global environment is seen as an economic phenomenon: environmental decisions are essentially economic ones. The idea that we should consider environmental consequences in economic decisions is

emphatically rejected, partly because it pays lip service to the environment; partly because environment invariably loses out; but really because, if a project is essentially flawed, it cannot be redeemed by environmental assessment, cost-benefit analysis, or environmental impact studies.

The most extreme version of this approach is summed up in the slogan, "the environment is the economy (stupid)." *All* economic decisions are environmental, and vice-versa—change one set of decisions and you will get exactly corresponding consequences for the other—both are expressions of a single type of decision, albeit expressed in different language, with different concerns and serving different interests.

Such theories have had a long, if obscure history. The nineteenth century Vermont thinker George Perkins Marsh demonstrated that global environmental degradation was the result of resource policies that undermined the productive basis of the earth. He was really the father of modern resource economics and "sustainable development." But it is hard to generate a popular movement out of such an arcane and technical version of the dismal science.

The Stockholm Declaration of 1972 discerned two issues, one of development and the other, environmental protection; it concerned itself with the relationship between the two. The Rio Declaration (1992) introduced the concept of sustainable development but, like Stockholm, concerned itself essentially with the relationship between these two concepts. Neither saw economic and environmental decisions as basically a single concept. Developing countries complained that environmental concerns amounted to a "new form of conditionality" imposed on the needs of development while environmentalists complained (somewhat less loudly) that environment was playing second fiddle to economic development. Meanwhile, armed with the World Trade Organization (WTO) Agreement of 1994, the transnational developers were laughing all the way to the World Bank.

While there was a great intellectual ferment in the '90s (in which the three authors were major players), it was not until *Natural Capitalism* appeared in 1999 that the third theory came into its own. It is based on the premise that the world is ridden *equally* with deep social and environmental problems and that they can be resolved only by the strategies of natural capitalism. These strategies are fourfold:

1. Radical Resource Productivity

Radically increased resource productivity will slow the depletion of the earth's natural resources; lower pollution, waste, and needless consumption; and provide the basis for worldwide full employment in meaningful jobs. About a quarter of U.S. $9 trillion GDP is wasted on unproductive use of resources, waste and human institutions that feed directly on the wasteful economy—prisons, security, avoidable or needless health care, wasteful transport systems, insurance costs, junk food, underemployment, social stress and breakdown among them. The authors demonstrate—entirely convincingly—that 90-95 percent reductions in materials and energy are currently possible in developed nations without diminishing quality of life, often with lower initial investment costs and invariably with greater rates of return.

2. Investing in Natural Capital

Worldwide planetary destruction can be reversed through reinvestment in sustaining, restoring, and expanding stocks of natural capital, so that the earth can produce more abundant natural resources with greater service value.

3. Biomimicry

The key to resource productivity is to reduce the wasteful "throughput" of materials by redesigning industrial systems on biological lines, enabling the constant low-energy reuse of materials in continuous closed cycles. There is no concept of waste in natural systems; nor need there be in human systems. And with the elimination of waste, we largely dismantle the "toxic economy."

4. The Service and Flow Economy

When these three concepts are extended into consumption, we see that they imply a shift from the conventional capitalist concept of a market for goods, for commodities. They shift to a concept of a market for *services*, since goods must be continuously reused, recycled, and "remanufactured" in order for the first three concepts to be applied in full. Producers, manufacturers, and marketers *must* provide a service; otherwise the concepts of natural capitalism cannot be (fully) applied. This is the thinking that lies behind the idea of "extended producer responsibility."

Expressed in such a summary form, without the wealth of detailed examples that the authors provide, it is hard to grasp what a radical and subversive theory *Natural Capitalism* puts forward. In traditional Marxist theory, capitalist exploitation takes the form of dirty and dangerous work: starvation wages; child labor, excessive hours, unemployment and all of the consequences such as bad sanitation, poor or non-existent housing, and pollution of the social environment. The key to social evil lies in capitalist *modes of production*, the way in which resources are mined, extracted, harvested, processed and manufactured. But *Natural Capitalism* goes beyond this. The causes of social and environmental breakdown are due almost entirely to the brute fact of the excessive and wasteful exploitation of natural resources—not to the modes of production.

The authors do not deny the effects of modes of production on human society. What they are saying is much deeper; it is the *fact* of resource exploitation and the industrial use of resources which gives rise to social and environmental devastation alike. For every high-paid resource sector worker, there are hundreds of others flipping hamburgers, incapacitated by environmental disease, or idle because of resource exhaustion, environmental devastation, and social breakdown.

But the four-fold strategies of natural capitalism do not cover everything. There is an age-old problem of political philosophy over the relationship between the usefulness of social projects and the way they are distributed in society—social justice. The idea that you can deduce the latter from the former has been discredited; we need two principles to underpin the good society, not one, and so we need some way of deciding whether a lot of social goods distributed among few people is better or worse than a smaller amount of goods distributed fairly and evenly among a wider group. We could place political leaders such as Ronald Reagan, Olaf Palme, and Fidel Castro on a spectrum as to how they viewed this dilemma; but the important thing is that there are two principles to consider and thus tensions between them.

So with *Natural Capitalism*. The authors are quire clear that the principles of natural capitalism alone cannot fulfill the socio-environmental project. We also need a principle of human capital or social justice that embraces such concepts as democratic systems of production and distribution of goods on the service-flow model; a distinct preference for fairness in distribution as opposed to "total dollar flow;" a realization that in pursuing natural capitalism, we have to redress inequities in global income and material well-being; and that natural capitalism will not succeed in anything but open, democratic societies.

This comes out clearly in the discussion of the environmentally benign Hypercar: without wholesale transport and land-use reform, the Hypercar could contribute to excessive automobility with effects on equity, urban structure, and social fabric. A clean hell to live and drive in is only marginally less bad than a dirty one.

Here lies the great flaw in the project of *Natural Capitalism*. The authors are clear that the problems and the solutions lie with private business. The next industrial revolution will be a transformation of conventional capitalism, not its demise in favor of eco-socialism. But the economy does not exist for the sake of business. Current industrial capitalism is described as a profitable, non-sustainable aberration in human development, which survives only because of its perverse accounting system. Current capitalism ignores the value of both human and natural capital, upon which its success depends.

With this harsh critique, we should expect the authors to promote a broad coalition of interests, such as progressive governments, environmentalists, social justice activists, and the labor movement to push, guide, and steer capitalism in the direction that is in the interests of everyone. On paper, they appear to do this. The frequent mention of the Just Transition Alliance and the discussions of green job creation for workers are especially welcome. But in the end we are left with pleas, exhortation, education, and appeals to financial self-interest directed toward business alone. Business people have always been Paul Hawken's main audience and the main clients of the two Lovins in their work on energy production and efficiency at the Rocky Mountain Institute in Colorado. The flaw is not that solutions lie in business operations—hard enough for any socialist to swallow—but that the keys to these solutions lie essentially with business alone. It is as if the authors have produced a powerful neo-Marxist program but without a theory of revolution to see it through!

Deep ecologists will not like the book because, while it aims for the integrity of natural systems, these are really instrumental in human purposes, which in turn depend for their realization on human artifice (technology). Those who believe that the information society itself comprises the next industrial revolution will also be disappointed. The authors are at pains to explain why digital technology does not amount to a social revolution (and they are right).

Nonetheless, *Natural Capitalism* is a huge achievement. Little is left out—the major omissions are in the areas of municipal operations, medical care and education, and the world's leading unsustainable industry, the military establishment. The authors are generous to those whose ideas they have adopted, such as Raymond Ayres, Janine Benyus, and Herman Daly. Benyus' work on biomimicry is highly original and plays a crucial part in the theory of natural capitalism. But the gray eminence behind *Natural Capitalism* is surely Herman Daly. We should all marvel at the sheer effort of intellect, perception, and imagination that led to the economic theory we now call "sustainable production."

To put down *Natural Capitalism* because of its omissions, dearth of strategy, or because we disagree with its politics would be a misguided and short-sighted mistake. The book will surely join *Silent Spring*, Herman Daly's *Steady-State Economics* (1991), and Paul Hawken's own *Ecology of Commerce* as the great environmental books of the later twentieth century.

PART VI

International Regimes in Health, Safety, and Environment

CHAPTER 12

Beware ISO

In the last decade, the International Organization for Standardization (ISO) has produced standards of corporate business performance in the areas of quality management of the production process and environmental management standards. The driving force behind this process is free trade. The first move is to treat substantive issues of working conditions and environmental protection merely as technical management problems, then to produce technical standards, then to incorporate them into international trade agreements so that they do not become "unnecessary obstacles to trade."

The purpose of this essay is to analyze the impact of these standards on working conditions and on environmental protection measures taken by businesses and governments.

BACKGROUND: THE ISO

The ISO was founded in 1946. For decades, the work of ISO consisted of generating a wide range of technical standards, such as those governing industrial equipment, health and safety devices, protective clothing, consumer items, signs and colors—anything, in fact, except electrotechnical activities (covered by the International Electrotechnical Commission) and pharmaceutical products (handled by the World Health Organization (WHO)).

Despite the fact that the ISO is often listed in the same breath as the WHO and the International Labour Organization (ILO), the ISO is not an agency of the United Nations (U.N.), nor is it, strictly speaking, an international governmental organization. Member bodies of the ISO are those "most representative of standardization" in the country and not all of these are governmental institutions or organizations incorporated by public law. Even where the member body is wholly public, it can still be business-dominated (see Section 2).

Beginning in 1987, the direction of ISO fundamentally changed, a trend which has attracted very little public attention. The first standards under the ISO 9000 Series on Quality Management appeared in that year and, unlike most of the previous work of ISO, they were concerned with policies, procedures, and activities in the workplace, and not merely with technical standards governing equipment, products, and devices. Work on the ISO 14000 Series on Environmental Management began in the 1990s as a result of public environmental concerns as expressed in the U.N. Conference on Environment and Development (UNCED) in 1992; but they would not have begun without the concern, essentially on the part of international business, that environmental pressures would impact on trade, and in particular on the new free trade regimes such as the General Agreement on Tariffs and Trade (the Uruguay Round of the GATT, 1994). In June 1996, the basic environmental management standards in the 14000 Series, together with the key standards on environmental auditing and certification, were formally adopted by the ISO. (Since the GATT legitimizes even draft standards, this is perhaps not much more than a formality!) The latest proposals for the ISO concern the development of sectoral standards (see Section 5) and the proposal to develop a Health and Safety Management Standard (see Section 6), even to the point of a whole new ISO 18000 Series on Health and Safety. Despite the fundamental shift from technical to policy standards, the term Technical Committee is used to cover the working bodies both of policy and of technical working groups.

2. NATIONAL STANDARDS BODIES AND THE ISO

We first have to understand how national standard-writing bodies relate to the work of ISO. Canada will serve as an example. Canada's member body at the ISO is the Standards Council of Canada (SCC), which governs the standard-making bodies in the country, or at least endorses the standards which they produce. (In other countries, the member body is often the National Safety Council, though the relationship between the national body and the ISO is not very different from that in Canada.) In practice, the body which contributes the most to the work of the ISO is the Canadian Standards Association (CSA). This body in turn is comprised of Technical Committees which frame technical standards. Labor and non-governmental organization (NGO) representation on the technical committees is often poor, mainly because of the expense of attending meetings, and it would in any case be impossible to match the business (or even the government) representation on these committees. And it is certainly true that some technical standards are of great political importance, such as the design of demand valves on breathing apparatus or calibration standards for gas detection equipment used in confined spaces. However, the main problem for the public interest is not the technical work of CSA, nor its implications for ISO, but in how the CSA is governed. On this, even Machiavelli would have thrown up his hands in despair. Here is a list of the governing bodies of CSA (readers may be able to add new ones, as they appear, apparently from nowhere, with alarming frequency):

- The Board of Directors;
- The Canadian Advisory Council (CAC);
- The Canadian Environmental Council (CEC);
- The Operating Committee of the CEC;
- The Environmental Steering Committee;
- The Health and Safety Strategic Steering Committee;
- The Priorities and Planning Committee; and
- The Standards Policy Board.

At the time of writing, ISO standards are adopted by the CAC.

In theory, constituency representation on CSA governing bodies (what the CSA calls a membership matrix) is designed to prevent the domination of CSA by any one party or interest. For instance, on the CEC, business is the biggest constituency; but it is outnumbered on paper by the combination of three others: government, professionals (for example, health professionals and technicians) and NGOs (including labor) [1]. For several reasons, this does not work. For one thing, there is not enough interest on the part of NGOs to fill all the slots and, on those that are filled, the members cannot usually afford to attend. Even if the slots were all filled and all the members present, all of the non-business representatives would have to vote as a bloc in order to defeat a business motion. This never happens, partly because the government representatives [2] vote with business and partly because many of the professionals work for, and are answerable to, business. In practice, there is usually a lone voice and a lone vote against any given motion, for example, from the Canadian Bar Association (over sectoral standards and the proposed Health and Safety Management Standard (Sections 5 and 6), business is divided).

Beyond the formalities, there are other irregularities. When challenged, a professional representative will change her/his affiliation (to business), and this is accepted by the Chair on the nod, without the consent of the member's sponsoring organization or the formal ratification of the CSA (which body would ratify, is another mystery). Some of the organizations listed as NGOs are nothing of the sort: they are consultants or bodies like the National Round Table on Environment and Economy. Some NGOs are listed when they are not members, while others are given voting status when they have accepted. membership only with observer status. Sometimes, faxed and proxy votes are accepted even though the vote may be for a revised resolution which the absent voters have never even seen!

All this palaver and chicanery is designed to disguise the CSA as a business-dominated organization. The fact is that the Canadian representatives on ISO Technical Committees are selected and sponsored by the CSA and most are business people. This is even more important when we bear in mind that, unlike a tripartite organization such as the ILO, the ISO has no mechanism for incorporating public or non-governmental participation into its activities.

Even if public interests wanted to participate in the work of ISO, they could not do so beyond a token or co-opting role in some advisory body or another. Engaging the ISO as a way of widening its legitimacy beyond its business orientation is not a practical possibility. Advice to anyone who wants to influence the direction of the ISO in some meaningful way is: don't even think about it. The ISO has to be influenced or fought from some other quarter, in some other forum or arena.

3. THE ISO 9000 SERIES ON QUALITY MANAGEMENT

The ISO 9000 Series comprises some 20 topic areas, including auditing and certification of product quality assurance. Quality Management under ISO is well-established in industrialized countries and all the propaganda points to the aim of establishing Quality Management as a pervasive world-wide system.

There are three sorts of possible threat posed by ISO 9000. The first is that it favors large organizations based in industrialized countries. A transnational corporation operating in a developing country will be able to meet ISO 9000 standards while its indigenous counterpart may not be able to do so, either because it does not have the management infrastructure or resources or because the mode of industrial organization does not fit with the dominant model. For instance, a textiles marketing co-operative will not be organized on the lines of companies with a charter of incorporation and a management hierarchy. The diversity, and not the standardization of the product, is the essence of such a business. Even the purchasing "system" may be quite haphazard, yet still effective in serving the needs of the organization. All this is the opposite of Quality Management.

The second sort of threat is to legislated consumer standards. Consumer product standards are of two sorts: the first an answer to the question, "how good, or reliable, or durable is the product?" and the second, "does the product do (well) what it is supposed to do?" The ISO 9000 does not cover the second question, leading to the joke (which is actually a serious point) that you can produce a concrete life jacket and still get certification under ISO 9000. But neither does ISO cover the first question; all that ISO 9000 does is to ensure that there are appropriate processes and procedures in place to assure Quality Management. For instance, a toy company could get certification under ISO 9000 when its products (notoriously) fall to bits as soon as they are used.

Despite the commonly used title "International Standards Organization," ISO 9000 does not, in fact, generate standards of product quality. All it does is to assess procedures; it does not even provide a measure or set of criteria whereby entirely different management systems are deemed to meet a common management standard. Thus, if ISO certification were used as a reason or occasion for allowing consumer standards to fall into abeyance, it would be disingenuous or fraudulent: consumer standards and ISO 9000 deal with entirely different things, and to hold up the latter as a substitute for the former would be entirely misleading. So far, there seem to be no concrete or obvious examples of this happening, but we should not be surprised to hear manufacturers of baby cribs or children's clothing claim an alibi in ISO 9000 certification.

The third threat is to workers' rights and interests in workplaces [3]. There are very few examples of ISO conformity procedures being handled by joint committees of workers and managers. The best that can be said is that some of the work on ISO conformity is done by employees who happen to be union members.

Managers may claim that

I. they need to know how specific skills are applied to materials and processes because ISO requires it;
ii. that workplace processes, procedures, and conditions have to be changed because ISO requires it; or
iii. that ISO overrides or cuts across the collective agreement.

None of these claims is correct and unless workers are aware of it, they will not have the tools to resist and fight back. The reason, again, is that ISO does not establish a standard whereby any given procedure can be judged in conformity or not. The question to be asked about the application of a specific skill is not "how is it effective?" but "does it work?"

Again, one way of realizing ISO 9000 is through Total Quality Management (TQM); but TQM is not required by ISO. Nor does a management procedure ever override the collective agreement. The theory behind collective bargaining, as expressed in industrial relations regimes, is that management has a wide area of exclusive decision known as management rights. To a greater or lesser degree, collective agreements made inroads into this preserve, bringing some areas under joint union-management control or under the control of workers. The true case is the opposite: where there is an apparent conflict between the requirements of ISO and a collective agreement, the latter always takes precedence. In the case of ISO, one aim should be to bring quality assurance under joint union-management oversight and control.

The moral of all this is that the threats posed by ISO 9000 are not in the existence of the series but in the way in which the items in it are used by employers and by governments.

4. THE ISO 14000 SERIES ON ENVIRONMENTAL MANAGEMENT

The international corporate agenda is to substitute voluntary international standards for mandatory national standards embodied in regulation [4]. Under free trade regimes, there are various ways in which systems of national regulation can be destroyed: business does not need voluntary international standards to destroy national regulations, but these are at least a useful alibi, an assurance that standards are still being met, in spite of the destruction of public institutions and the decay of national government.

In the area of environmental protection and ecosystem integrity, the chosen vehicle for realizing and implementing international standards is the ISO. The ISO 14000 Series is a large range of "standards," including the basic environmental management system documents on guidance and specification (ISO 14000-14004); environmental auditing and certification (ISO 14010-14015); environmental performance (ISO 14031); life cycle assessment (ISO 14041-14044); environmental labeling (ISO 14020-14024); and environmental aspects of product standards (ISO 14060).

As an institution (despite the peculiarities of ISO, noted above), the organization is recognized and institutionalized in free trade agreements. Annex 3 of the GATT Agreement on Technical Barriers to Trade (TBT) is a Code of Practice for the Preparation, Adoption, and Application of Standards. In this, as in the TBT Agreement, ISO is named and recognized. Standardizing bodies in member states must notify the ISO/IEC Information Centre in Geneva if they accept or withdraw from the Code. Under the Code, member states have to send periodic reports to ISONET about their standardizing activities. In TBT, member states must give preference to international standards wherever feasible. The implication is that by adopting international standards, including those of the ISO, they would not be "creating unnecessary obstacles to international trade." Further, a standard can involve "production methods," thus covering policy and procedural standards, such as ISO 9000 and ISO 14000.

The GATT Agreement on TBT is enshrined in the North American Free Trade Agreement (NAFTA) (Art. 903), as is the primacy accorded to international standards (Art. 905). Further, unlike the GATT, ISO is specifically included in NAFTA as an "international standardizing body" (Art. 915). The definition of a standard in NAFTA includes an "operating method," making it clear that policy and procedural standards, such as ISO 9000 and ISO 14000 are included, as well as strictly technical standards.

While ISO 9000 and ISO 14000 are not specifically enshrined in the GATT (unlike, say, the standards of the Codex Alimentarius Commission), they clearly count as the sort of standard that could be used in evidence in trade challenge cases. In particular, a business that was certified under ISO 14000 would be virtually immune from any accusation that its environmental practices constituted an obstacle to trade. On a more mundane level, one of the listed advantages of an effective environmental management system (EMS) is that it ensures customers of commitment to demonstrable environmental management (ISO 14004, 0.2), that is, that it serves to deflect detailed inquiries about environmental performance. Ironically, neither the goals of free trade nor of environmental protection are listed among the benefits.

APPLICATION OF ISO

There are two key things to understand about the application of ISO. The first is that it does not establish a standard of environmental protection, nor does it measure environmental performance. Environmental performance is not audited, nor is there any cross-referencing between the auditing standards and the environmental performance standard, which does not in any case measure environmental performance or evaluate the record of the enterprise against tangible criteria. Second, ISO 14000 does not measure or audit compliance with environmental regulations. To be sure, the organization's EMS must have an environmental policy, which includes "a commitment to comply with relevant environmental legislation and regulations . . ." (ISO 14001, 4.1). But this is not a requirement for certification under ISO 14000, nor is compliance audited. That ISO 14000 does not measure compliance is acknowledged in the documentation: "It should be noted that this standard does not establish absolute requirements for environmental performance beyond commitment, in the policy, to compliance with applicable legislation and regulations and to continual improvement. Thus, two organizations carrying out similar activities but having different environmental performance may both comply with its requirements" (ISO 14001, Introduction).

The danger of ISO 14000 is that the Series will be used as a surrogate for compliance with environmental laws. For instance, it already has been proposed that companies certified under ISO 14000 will get a "holiday" from the enforcement of regulations, even though ISO 14000 has nothing to do with compliance, nor the company's compliance records [5]. Regulations which remain on the books but which are unenforced are useless, a form of de facto deregulation.

This process would be further legitimized by referencing ISO standards in legislation. There is provision for this in Bill C-25, the Regulations Act, now before the Canadian Parliament. The House of Commons Standing Committee on Environment and Sustainable Development recommended (June 1995) that ISO 14000 be referenced in legislation governing "federal entities," specifically those covered in Part IV of the Canadian Environmental Protection Act (CEPA). The ISO 14000 already has been referenced in forest sector legislation in Ontario.

Most businesses would have no problem with this, since they support ISO and since, to all intents and purposes, the standards remain "voluntary;" they have no regulatory force. Policy standards are difficult and time-consuming for governments to enforce and, in any case, it is impossible in legal practice for governments to prosecute in the event of violation of a policy standard. The threat of prosecution (rather than the actual number of prosecutions) is the chief incentive for compliance with a legislated standard or regulation. When we combine these factors with the real possibility of de facto deregulation, the dangers of referencing ISO standards in legislation are obvious. (It is unlikely that ISO certification would generally be required by law.)

There is, however, one concern that businesses have over ISO standards and that is the "double burden" of carrying out the onerous task of obtaining ISO certification and of complying with national regulations. Since businesses perceive it to be in their interests to do the former, they are likely to want to escape or evade the latter. Considerations such as this have led some businesses to oppose the development of an ISO Health and Safety Management Standard (Section 6). But to claim that there is a context of "increasingly stringent legislation" (ISO 14010 Introduction) is simply not true.

The conclusion of this section is that there is nothing objectionable in the existence of 14000: everything depends on how the documents are used politically by employers and by the governments who are beholden to them. If in addition to its impact on national environmental regulation, ISO 14000 were held up as sufficient for environmental protection in free trade agreements, this would have the effect of nullifying attempts to have international environmental agreements override the GATT. Environmental management procedures would be substituted for tangible international environmental protection measures.

5. ISO SECTORAL STANDARDS

There are proposals to develop ISO sectoral standards, particularly in the area of forest management and forest products. The argument is that some sectors face specific problems and areas of economic activity which cannot be addressed by general ISO standards, and that the needed business credibility will not be secured simply by conforming to the general industrial norms.

Some segments of business oppose these moves. They fear that there will be a proliferation of sectoral standards with a confusing burden of having to conform both to some of the general standards and all of the sector-specific ones; they fear that sectoral standards will be more stringent than the general norms, so that their own sector will face an artificially high and unfair burden of compliance [6].

Currently, Canada (through the CSA) will support a "bridging document" on Forestry in regard to ISO 14001 on EMS. This is known as the "New Zealand Process" and Canada will support a "Type III Technical Report of ISO." Where the standard would go after this is not clear: it could constitute a formal ISO sectoral standard in ISO 14000, a freestanding ISO standard, a guideline (comparable to ISO 14004), or it could simply go nowhere.

Quite apart from any programmatical objection to ISO (the theme of this chapter), there is one nagging doubt that has been expressed by business as well as by critics of ISO. The aim of the forest sector is to attain a degree of credibility about its forest practices so that governments, consumers, and customers do not discriminate against their products. Although draft standards envisaged in this sector may contain more (that is, sector-specific) parameters than the general EMSs, they are no different from the general norm in that they do not comprise a standard of corporate environmental behavior, nor do they measure performance or compliance. "Given that TC 207 [ISO Technical Committee 207] has no mandate to develop standards prescribing performance, any management standard developed within TC 207 will not satisfy needs that are performance-oriented" [7].

What is ominous is that, in the light of the opening discussion in this section, ISO Forest Management Certification may make it unlawful for governments and businesses to discriminate against products from companies certified under the standard. So we would get the worst of both worlds: no improvement through ISO of forest practices and the entrenchment in international law of the non-standards of the ISO.

This gives rise to an important issue which is both controversial and obscure. It concerns the role in international trade of standards set by environmental non-governmental organizations (ENGOs) such as the Forest Stewardship Council (FSC). The question is: is a standard set by an international ENGO and which is adopted as a trading requirement by businesses or governments a legitimate term of trade or is it a trade barrier, an "unnecessary obstacle to international trade?"

COMPLICATING FACTORS

The issue is complicated by a number of factors. The first is that there is an irregularity in free trade agreements. The parties to such agreements are national governments but the bodies which write standards are often "non-governmental." In the GATT, member governments must take reasonable measures to ensure that non-governmental bodies conform to the terms of the treaty (TBT, Art. 8). The NAFTA is similar but more detailed (Ch. 9). However, the "non-governmental standardizing bodies" clearly mean the ISO and the corresponding national organizations. The treaties did not envisage a role for ENGOs such as the FSC. On paper, there seems to be nothing to prevent the FSC from registering with the ISO/IEC Information Centre in Geneva, though bodies subscribing to the Code of Practice are referred to as national or regional, not international.

The second complicating factor is that standards in free trade agreements are always referred to as "technical" whereas, as we have seen, some ISO standards relate to policies and procedures yet (misleadingly) still fall under the heading "technical." If ISO policy standards fall under the GATT, then so should those of the FSC. Nor do ISO environmental management standards and the (regional) forest practices standards of the FSC overlap, since the latter set tangible standards of environmental practice while ISO 14000 deals, essentially, only with management procedures. It would be hard to make out a case for duplication, something that World Trade Organization (WTO) members must try to avoid.

Thus, there seems to be no reason why both ISO and FSC standards could not be adopted internationally, without creating barriers to trade. Environmentalists, for their part, fear that an ISO sectoral standard would pre-empt those of the FSC, ruling them out as an unnecessary obstacle to trade. Arguably, the best strategy would be for FSC to attempt to attain status in the GATT, since an ISO sectoral standard is quite a long way off.

In general, there are three sorts of rules governing international trade transactions:

I. rules over what businesses may buy and sell from each other;
ii. national import-export rules; and
iii. rules over government procurement of goods and services.

There are few rules of the first sort other than the obligation to abide by commercial contracts, though businesses are constrained by rules over labeling (the proposed ISO 1420-24 rules on environmental labeling will become highly relevant), by national bans and restrictions on hazardous products, and by import-export rules. The thrust of the GATT is to limit the number and scope of such rules as much as possible, except where they positively promote free trade, as—it is claimed—do ISO 9000 and 14000. The rules over procurement are different, since the parties are of course governments, not businesses. The GATT TBT rules do not apply to government procurement; instead, there is a separate Agreement on Government Procurement (Marrakesh, 15 April 1994), accession to which is optional among WTO member countries. However, the language of Art. 6, Technical Specifications, is similar to the TBT Chapter, implying that governments would be in a similar position to private businesses when it comes to citing international standards such as those of the ISO and the FSC.

6. THE PROPOSED ISO HEALTH AND SAFETY MANAGEMENT STANDARD

Health and safety is not addressed in ISO 14000 though the standard "does not seek to discourage an organization from developing integration of such management system elements" (ISO 14001, Introduction). Health and safety requirements are not certified under ISO 14000.

Support for ISO work in this area is not strongly or universally supported by businesses [8]. The main pressure comes from health and safety professionals, some of whom have lost status and employment due to business and government downsizing or who have lost jobs due to the collapse of the health and safety enforcement system (as has happened in Ontario). Registration, auditing, and certification would be done by these same underemployed professionals.

The strategy is similar to that which is being employed by the Canadian forest industry. National centers move to produce their own management systems, which are then put forward (usually in draft form) to the international body for consideration as the basis for an international standard.

The response from most of the labor movement has been to oppose the development by ISO of work in this area, to express some strong skepticism about the project, or to lay down conditions both for what should be in the standard and for the terms of reference of the project, which would determine whether labor would participate in the project.

There is one fundamental difference between ISO policy standards to date and the health and safety proposal. In the area of environmental protection, we can make a clear distinction between environmental management and environmental performance. It is the confusion or confounding of these two in the way that ISO 14000 is used or applied, which is the root cause of the threat to environmental protection regimes. In health and safety, we cannot do this. The way that health and safety has developed internationally as a discipline involves:

a) the development of health and safety standards at the national and international levels through tripartite consultations between workers, employers, and governments;

b) the exercise of health and safety in the workplace through bipartite institutions and operations such as joint health and safety committees or work councils;

c) worker' rights, such as the right to refuse unsafe work, the right to participate (for example, joint committees), plus the right to information and training;

d) the obligation of employers to conform to a series of legislated rules, including rules governing workers' rights; and

e) the existence of a dedicated health and safety government infrastructure, with a system of enforcement and compliance, backed by a health and safety inspectorate.

All of these concepts are to be found in ILO Convention No. 155, the generic Occupational Health and Safety Convention, 1981. This means that either health and safety is not a management function at all (and thus not the sort of thing that ISO management standards can accommodate) or the standard would have to include considerations which have deliberately been excluded from all other ISO policy standards to date. Faced with the double burden of dealing with a (so-far) entrenched health and safety system and the demands of ISO certification, it is no wonder that some employers have opposed the ISO getting into this area at all.

The chief danger for labor, however, is that an ISO Health and Safety Management Standard would come to be used as an empty surrogate for the health and safety regimes which have been built up over a century of carnage and campaigning and which were implemented in detail from roughly the early 1970s onwards. Health and safety as merely a management function would cut workers out of the action completely and produce workplace conditions and procedures entirely alien to the regimes of the last quarter century.

An ISO workshop on the proposal was held in Geneva in 1996. The labor group at the workshop was led by the International Confederation of Free Trade Unions (ICFTU) [9]. While governments took a mainly neutral position, labor, business, and (interestingly) the insurance industry were on the whole opposed. It is therefore unlikely that the ISO will proceed to develop a Health and Safety Management Standard. However, there are likely to be moves to begin work on a Guideline as an alternative to a standard. This could be a move to write a standard via the back door: experience at the national level indicates that Guidelines become standards, with auditing and certification, despite disclaimers that Guidelines should not be used in this way.

CONCLUSION

The thrust of this article has been to demonstrate that there is little problem over the existence of ISO management standards in themselves. Rather, the issue is the role they play in "global governance." The first flaw in the process of developing international standards is to treat substantive issues of workplace democracy, working conditions, and environmental protection merely as technical issues of process management. When the standards are enshrined in international law, they then become a substitute for tangible national regulations (national standards) and, possibly also, substantive international agreements (treaties, conventions, and protocols). And insofar as developing countries do not have effective national regulations, the temptation is to look to ISO for standards of corporate behavior, which could well impede the development of effective regulations to protect workers and the environment.

The work of ISO is an aspect of business advocacy of "voluntary standards" as opposed to hard regulation. So far, it is succeeding. National systems of regulation remain the most effective ways to protect working conditions and the environment: they stand in need of restoration and advancement. How to prevent ISO-GATT-WTO from subverting this progressive agenda is less clear.

NOTES

1. The Canadian Labour Congress put forward two proposals on environmental auditing in the ISO 14000 series for adoption as the Canadian position in the ISO TC 207. The first proposal was:

    "Where by law, agreement or workplace practice, the employer is obliged to consult with employees over conditions of work, the employer shall consult with workers, or their representatives, over the conduct of the audit, from planning to conclusion."

    This was the position that the ICFTU has argued for in the consultations that led to Agenda 21 of the UNCED Conference in Rio, June 1992.

    The second proposal was that, among the topics to be covered in an audit are natural resource input conservation; pollution prevention and waste (generation) reduction; energy efficiency and waste management and recycling. In other words, there had to be hard "external" criteria for environmental audits.

    Both proposals were rejected by CSA, the first on the curious grounds that if this were national practice, it would be done anyway, ISO or not. As it stands, there are no "external" criteria in ISO audits; criteria for particular audits are drawn up by agreement between the company and the auditor. It is not too much of an exaggeration to say that the content of an audit is decided by the company being audited!

Of just as much importance is the fact that the CSA did not know what to do with a proposal which came from outside the business orbit. The proposals were sent to the relevant CSA Technical Committee, which sent them back to the CSA Environmental Council with a rejection slip. The appropriate policy-setting body, the CSA Environmental Council, had no say in the matter.

2. In free trade agreements, governments must take reasonable measures to ensure that standard-writing bodies conform to the trade treaties. In the CSA, they have not used this sort of power. For instance, it is Canadian policy (Government of Canada, Pollution Prevention, A Federal Strategy for Action, July 1995) to incorporate pollution prevention into international standards. While there is evidence that the Canadian government raised the issue with the CSA, it did not pursue the issue at the CSA Environmental Council nor did it seek the support of other parties in pushing the issue to a vote. Not that it would have made much difference: the Canadian government's definition of pollution prevention is progressive and constructive; but the ISO's definition is so vague and all-inclusive that a commitment to pollution prevention is really a commitment to the status quo, "we are doing it already" (ISO 14000.3.13). In this episode, the Canadian Government was reduced to asking the permission of business to implement its own official policies—and was turned down.

3. The ISO 9000 and its ramifications have been well analyzed in "ISO 9000: An Examination of the Labour Issues in the Implementation of ISO 9000 Certification," by John Anderson with material by Jonathan Eaton, April, 1995.

4. This point is made, as a passing observation in "ISO Inside Out, ISO and Environmental Management," by Pierre Hauselmann; A WWF International Discussion Paper, August 1996.

A somewhat different line of argument is taken in "ISO 14001: An Uncommon Perspective, Five Public Policy Questions for Proponents of the ISO 14000 Series" by Benchmark Environmental Consulting, for the European Environment Bureau, Revised, November 1995. This paper argues that, though ISO 14000 is an international standard, it does nothing to ensure conformity to international environmental standards and regimes. True enough: but the only tangible standards so far are (roughly) those contained in the Montreal Protocol for ozone depletion and the Basel Convention on the transport of hazardous waste. The rest are only vague declarations of intent. More important is the failure of the ISO 14000 series to assess compliance with national environmental protection regimes. These are admittedly uneven; though only these alone do anything much to regulate corporate environmental performance.

The paper goes on to commend those organizations which have committed themselves to uniform standards in their transnational operations, including the Canadian Chemical Producers Association. Whether such organizations deserve such commendation is highly dubious. See D. Bennett, "The Canadian Chemical Polluters' Association?" (unpublished MS, 1996), where it has been argued that the CCPA has been very successful in international image-making while pursuing an agenda of national deregulation with a vengeance.

5. See "Rethinking Environmental Regulatory Implementation: Interim Report" (for Discussion Purposes Only), Environment Canada, 1996, pages 16-26).

6. See the Submission by Imperial Oil Limited on the Sustainable Forest Management Standard, to the CSA-CEC, 1995.
7. Imperial Oil, op cit., page 2.
8. Business has contended that, far from facilitating trade, a Health and Safety Management Standard would become a trade barrier, since many businesses would be unable to meet the standard. This argument is equally applicable to ISO 9000 and 14000, an avenue which businesses prefer not to explore. It is possible, however, that businesses are now having second thoughts about the whole range of ISO policy standards: there are far too many of them and they are open to abuse, in view of widespread reports of companies "buying" ISO 9000 certification in the United States.
9. At the International Workshop on Occupational Health and Safety Management Systems Standardization, an ISO Contribution?, the labor presentations were given by Bruno Zwingmann (DGB, Germany); Ken-Ichi Kumagai (JTUC-Rengo, Japan); James S. Frederick (USWA for the AFL-CIO, U.S.A.); Pascal Etienne (IN-PACT, France); Tom Mellish (TUC, U.K.); Marc Sapir (TUTB-ETUC, for the ICFTU); and Dave Bennett (CLC-Canada). At a similar workshop in Toronto in May 1996 organized by the Standards Council of Canada, the labor presentation on behalf of the CLC was given by Anthony Pizzino (CUPE). The Canadian delegation at Geneva was organized by the Standards Council of Canada, which opposed the development of a Health and Safety Management Standard by ISO.

Though the labor movement generally opposes the development of an ISO Health and Safety Standard, some unions take the position that management standards, including certification standards, should include working conditions and social criteria. The International Federation of Building and Woodworkers, for instance, advocates the inclusion of such considerations in all relevant standards, whatever the sponsoring body, such as ISO or FSC.

CHAPTER 13

ISO and the WTO:
A Report to the International Confederation of Free Trade Unions' Working Party on Health, Safety, and Environment

In this Report:

- Why is ISO important?
- Developments in the ISO 14000 Environmental Management Series
- The Case of ISO 14020 Environmental Labeling Standards
- Comparison of ISO 14020 with the Biosafety Protocol
- The Proposed ISO Health and Safety Management Standard: A Defeat for Globalization

1. Why is ISO Important?

The International Organization for Standardization (ISO) generates, among other standards, a series of management standards, particularly the ISO 9000 series on Quality Management and the ISO 14000 series on Environmental Management. Like all other ISO standards, these are referred to as "technical standards" though there is really nothing technical about them.

ISO standards are developed by committees and working groups comprised of national standard-writing bodies, which in turn are comprised of business representatives, government personnel and professional management personnel, often again employed by private business. The ISO 14000 series is developed by Technical Committee (TC) 207.

Under the World Trade Organization (WTO) Agreement (1994), Members (governments) are obliged to adopt international standards wherever feasible and this includes ISO standards. One consequence is that businesses (including governments as trading parties) can make adherence or certification/registration under ISO standards a term or condition of trade with a foreign business. Thus, the intended result is that we will have a globally harmonized management system in which there are no barriers to international trade in the form of national standards diverging from the international norms.

The unofficial business agenda is more important than this official one. ISO standards are known as "voluntary standards" whether or not they are adopted or referenced in national laws and whether or not they are formally adopted by national standard-writing bodies, which are themselves "voluntary" (non-governmental) organizations. The aim of some transnational corporations and trade associations is to have adoption by business of management standards remove the need for national regulations, in the name of "voluntary standards" or voluntary compliance. The WTO Agreement (and NAFTA, 1994) puts very severe constraints on the ability of governments to regulate, for example, environmental protection. The unofficial agenda is thus one of deregulation in which voluntary management standards are the surrogate for national regulations. Provided a business is properly managed, the environment will be taken care of, without regulation.

The role of international voluntary standards is part of a wider business agenda which in theory accords a place for international treaties and Conventions. In practice, international treaties: 1) cover relatively small areas of environmental protection and sustainable development; 2) they are hard to enforce; and 3) they are always liable to succumb to WTO rules, challenges, and dispute procedures.

The unofficial agenda of deregulation puts public interest groups in a dilemma. On the face of it, there is very little in the management standards that anyone could quarrel with. It is not the content of the standards but their role in the global political economy which subverts the public interest. This being so, some public interest groups have tried to influence ISO, for example, by working through national delegations to ISO or by participation at the international level by groups acting in their own right, for example, The World Wildlife Fund for Nature (WWF International).

The merit of these ventures is dubious. First, ISO accords no place to the public interest in its consultation structures. The balance is tilted strongly against NGOs. Second, paradoxically, the significant strengthening of ISO standards only makes them more convincing as a surrogate for regulation and would thus serve the deregulation agenda, which is the last thing that a real public interest group would want. But, finally, there are structural reasons which, as we will soon see, prevent ISO standards from being strengthened in socially significant ways.

2. Developments in the ISO 14000 Environmental Management Series

The ISO 9000 Quality Management Series is under review. Also under review is the relationship between ISO 9000 and ISO 14000, with a view to joint certification for environmental and quality management. Although ISO 14000 has not quite been finalized, it too is now under review. We should really regard all ISO management standards as under a revolving review: the WTO Agreement legitimizes even draft standards.

The main ISO 14000 standards are in series as follows:

ISO 14000: guidance and specification
ISO 14010: environmental auditing and certification
ISO 14020: environmental labeling
ISO 14030: environmental performance
ISO 14040: life cycle assessment.

Though the review of ISO 14000 may result in some changes, it is unlikely to achieve anything significant. The reason is that the terms of reference of TC 207 preclude ISO 14000 from laying down "performance requirements," that is, they do not prescribe what *must* be achieved or implemented as a test of adherence or certification. Many standards, for example, ISO 14031 on environmental performance evaluation, suggest a range of criteria to be considered when assessing performance, but they all stop short of requiring them. In particular, compliance with environmental laws is not a mandatory test in environmental certification exercises, nor are there any mandatory environmental norms, such as Pollution Prevention, energy use reduction, resource conservation, "throughput" reduction per unit of product, or eco-efficiency. The situation will remain as it always has been: a well-managed enterprise but no clue as to whether it meets any environmental standards worth the name.

3. The Case of ISO 14020, Environmental Labeling

The ISO 14020 series is rather different from the rest; it lays down the sort of language which is permitted or prohibited on eco-labels—both self-declared environmental claims and statements by third parties, for example, eco-logo certification bodies, for all *non-food* items.

There are numerous business objections to ISO 14020, not all of them coherent and consistent with each other:

a) voluntary standards should have no legal force;
b) voluntary standards should not be prescriptive—to the extent that ISO 14020 rules out certain language from eco-labels it is in a small way prescriptive;
c) eco-labels can contain reference to Process and Production Methods (PPMs) since the environmental impact of a product concerns its origin and method of production as well as its use and disposal; and so
d) ISO 14020 is a potential barrier to trade

To the objection that ISO standards should have no legal force, they are clearly enshrined in the WTO Agreement and, to that extent, they form part of international trade law. Second, to the objection that ISO standards should not be prescriptive, it can be said that there is no contradiction between a standard that is voluntary but which contains mandatory elements; "if (but only if) you adhere to such-and-such a standard, there are certain things you must do. . . ." There is thus confusion between a non-binding standard and what specifics, if any, follow from its adoption. It is quite true that ISO 14020 is prescriptive; whether it contradicts the terms of reference of TC 207 is another matter. As to whether ISO 14020 is a potential barrier to trade, it quite clearly lays down restrictions on all trading parties, but then environmental auditing and certification requirements can do the same—if companies insist on them as terms of trade.

The question of ISO 14020 and PPMs touches a nerve. In the WTO Agreement, no Member can discriminate against traded goods on grounds of PPMs, for example, products made with child labor or under sweatshop conditions, Member governments must also try to frame their regulations without references to PPMs. ISO 14020 conflicts with the spirit of the WTO Agreement in that it allows references to PPMs on labels. For instance, a producer of genetically modified cotton could claim on the label that no chemical pesticides were used in its production and that (therefore) the product is beneficial to the environment. All that ISO 14020 requires is that such claims be environmentally relevant, specific, and verifiable. A more obvious reference to PPMs is "made from recycled materials."

WTO members must still not discriminate against genetically modified cotton but the mere fact that PPMs can appear on eco-labels is a small chink in the armor of the WTO, enabling consumers to make informed choices about genetically modified organisms (GMOs) in non-food products.

4. Comparison of ISO 14020 with the Biosafety Protocol

The Cartahena Protocol to the UN Convention on Biodiversity (1992), negotiated in Montreal, Canada in January 2000, regulates trade in items containing genetically modified organisms (GMOs). The Protocol conflicts with the WTO Agreement in several significant ways. Among them: Parties (governments) are allowed to discriminate against GMO items, for example, they can refuse them entry, on grounds of the PPMs used in the product—despite the claim of the producers that the items are "substantially equivalent" to non-GMO products. Secondly, some traded GMO items must be labeled as such. This goes much further than ISO 14020, which only permits (non-food) GMOs to be labeled, and then only in environmentally relevant ways. Whether the Cartahena Protocol will successfully override the WTO Agreement in practice is an open question. On paper, it is a breakthrough.

5. The Proposed ISO Health and Safety Management Standard; A Defeat for Globalization

Early in 1997, ISO decided against beginning work on a workplace health and safety management standard. There was an understanding that the International Labour Organization (ILO) would begin work on a health and safety management system through its tripartite structure, which gives equal representation to labor, business, and member governments. Yet in 1999, the British employers, abetted by health and safety professionals in the British Standards Institution, began a move to revive the work of ISO on health and safety management systems.

Thanks to intensive and pervasive organizing efforts by the ICFTU, this move was narrowly defeated in April 2000. It is true that some national health and safety management standards accord with the principles expressed in ILO Convention No. 155 (1981) Concerning Occupational Safety and Health. But there was no reason whatsoever to think that this would be true of an international standard emanating from ISO. None of the existing ISO management standards requires compliance with legislation; none of them involve workers in decision-making; and none of them have seen the health of workers as an essential part of sustainable development. There is every reason to believe that workers would have been written out of workplace governance completely, with health and safety audits, undertaken solely by managers, replacing both worker participation and government inspections.

The ILO Draft Guidelines on Occupational Safety and Health Management Systems (OSH—MS, Draft of 15-04-2000), by contrast, embodies principles that have been part of health and safety for at least a generation. The effect of an ISO standard would have been to eradicate these principles from the practice of health and safety and turn it into a mere line management function, without government intervention, without worker participation and with no place for worker health as a social value standing in the way of profit and free enterprise.

To the extent that ISO has again been kept out of health and safety, this represents a major victory for the public interest. One aim of globalization is to bring every area of economic activity under WTO rules. As in the case of the Multilateral Agreement on Investment (MAI), this move in health and safety has so far been defeated.

SOURCES

D. Bennett, Beware ISO, *New Solutions, 7*:3, Spring 1997.
J. Tickner, ISO 14000: Will It Deter Cleaner Production? *New Solutions, 8*:3, 1998.

Note: The International Labour Organization formally adopted its Guidelines on Occupational Safety and Health Management Systems in June 2001.

CHAPTER 14

Health and Safety Management Systems: Liability or Asset?

THE ILO SAFETY AND HEALTH MANAGEMENT GUIDELINES

In the spring of 2001, the International Labour Organization endorsed its Guidelines on Safety and Health Management Systems. The Guidelines have their background in several national models in the area of what are known as "voluntary standards"; some of these will be examined in due course. But in order to understand the ILO Guidelines, we have to understand the organization itself.

The ILO was founded in 1919 as an agency of the League of Nations; it was the only organization of the League to survive into the era of the United Nations as its oldest agency. The ILO is unique in another way. It is the only agency of the UN which is run by parties in addition to national governments. Thus the ILO is governed by a body comprised equally of representatives of employers, governments, and workers. This tripartite governance extends into the development of the ILO's "instruments" such as Conventions, Recommendations, Codes of Practice and Guidelines; even Guidelines are developed on a tripartite basis and are endorsed by the ILO governing bodies [1]. Though some basic rules of industrial relations have to be endorsed by member countries as a condition of membership of the ILO, acceptance of ILO instruments is voluntary. In the case of Codes of Practice and Guidelines there is no formal procedure of national acceptance.

The Safety and Health Management System Guidelines require a translation of their content into a "national system." Where this is done, it is accomplished normally not by the government but by the national "standard-writing body" as a "voluntary standard." This does not preclude the adoption or referencing of the voluntary standard in legislation, though in the case of management standards generally, this is rarely done.

The voluntary acceptance of ILO instruments means that, as such, there is nothing to require a nation to adopt them. Further, the enforcement tools available to the ILO to pressure a country to fulfill its commitments, once an instrument has been ratified, are very limited. Workers are the chief beneficiaries of the work of the ILO, so it is organized workers who have to work the hardest to ensure that their rights and employment standards are implemented and respected.

This is true of the rights and powers embodied in the Safety and Health Management Guidelines. The first thing to be said about the Guidelines is that they differ from previous models in one essential respect: they embody the rights, perspectives, and experiences of workers. Workers are an equal partner or player with management in devising and carrying out measures to protect their health and safety; they are participants in securing their own health and safety. After all, it is not management's health and safety that is at risk but the workers' health and safety. "Workers are not objects to be managed, like machines or other factors of production. They are living, breathing, thinking human beings who have the most fundamental stake in any system of health and safety that affects their workplace. They must be involved at the workplace level up to and including any international consensus standard" [2].

The ILO Guidelines are in three parts: a short section on objectives; a rather longer section on translating the Guidelines into national practice; and, a long section on "The OSH management system in the organization" (i.e., the workplace). The opening sections make it clear that the ILO management system is one approach or a "practical tool" for assisting the parties in the workplace (mainly, but not only, workers, their representatives, and management) in fulfilling health and safety duties in the organization of the workplace. The long section on the management system in the organization (the workplace) is comprised of 21 topics, including the employer's OSH policy; workers' participation; responsibility and accountability; training; system planning; OSH objectives; hazard prevention; performance monitoring and measurement; health and safety investigations; audits; management review; preventive and corrective action; and continual improvement.

This listing is exhaustive and much more comprehensive than national models. It is however a curiosity. Virtually all national systems contain such lists and they contain them at the expense of any description or prescription of what a workplace management system looks like, how it is structured, how it functions, how it relates to the management of the enterprise generally, how it is reconciled with the functions and responsibilities of other parties. There is no discussion of key management roles or reporting relationships. Anyone who looks to management system models for clues as to how managements work or could work in relation to health and safety will be disappointed. Health and safety professionals have, in a sense, created their own mystery.

The ILO Guidelines have several distinctive features, which become relevant when they are contrasted with previous models.

1. The all-important question of *worker participation,* discussed above. No national model comes close to the ILO Guidelines in requiring worker participation.

2. *Legal Compliance.* The ILO Guidelines make it clear that compliance with health and safety laws and regulations is an essential management function and required by any party that adopts the Guidelines. By contrast, legal compliance is either not required or is not a prominent part of national management systems. The rationale—or the excuse—for such a void is that compliance engenders a mentality of minimum standards and so militates against the notion of continual improvement.

3. *Hazard versus risk.* In the ILO Guidelines, the term "hazard" is sometimes used, at other times "risk," and yet other times "hazard or risk" in an attempt to balance the two notions. The reason for this is the wholesale rush to risk assessment as the precondition of taking any form of action in regard to health and safety [3]. Risk assessment is perceived by some as a permissive technique which either results in minimal action or which endorses the status quo on the grounds that the risk to health is negligible or "manageable." By contrast, the identification of a hazard, along with a precautionary approach, is held to be good and sufficient reason for intervention or action, either by way of prevention measures or controls. Hence, a motive of some who developed the Guidelines was to balance the notion of risk with that of hazard. By contrast, some national models such as the British read more like a treatise on risk assessment than on management systems, even though, strictly speaking, the technique of risk assessment has no essential connection whatever to a management system, except in the pernicious sense of "managing risks."

4. *Specification versus Performance Standards.* Most national systems are performance standards in the sense that managers and auditors have a wide range of discretion as to what they have to do to meet the standards embodied in the documentation. They are also performance standards in that specific objectives are rarely specified. Instead, there are tests like whether the system allows the employers' health and safety policies to be realized, which begs the question of whether such policies are themselves useful or efficacious in promoting workplace health and safety. In other words, there are no clear criteria by which health and safety performance can be judged. The ILO Guidelines, by contrast, contain specific objectives which have to be measured to demonstrate conformity to the standard. The rationale—or excuse—for performance standards is that having a management system is embodied in a "voluntary standard" and therefore nothing can be required or mandatory. This is a fallacy: the fact that something is voluntary does not mean that, if it is accepted, there can be no items which have to be adopted in order to conform to it.

5. *Audits.* All health and safety management systems have a provision for periodic audits. These may be "external" or "internal" to the organization; when they are "external," there may also be certification or "registration" as a putative guarantee that the audit has been conducted properly. (The ILO Guidelines are neutral as to whether audits are internal or external and there is no requirement for certification.) But the content of the audits is rarely specific, again giving wide discretion as to what is audited and how the audit is conducted. The ILO Guidelines, by contrast, are quite specific over the content, the procedure and the objectives of audits.

In the ILO Guidelines, it is not the *system* that is audited but the system in relation to health and safety performance: audits are to determine whether the 21 elements of the system (or a sub-set) are in place, adequate, and effective in protecting the health and safety of workers and in preventing incidents. Among the specific objectives of an audit are a determination of whether the management system is effective in promoting full workers' participation; whether the system responds to previous performance evaluations and audits; whether the organization achieves legal compliance; and whether the system fulfills the goals of continual improvement and best OSH practice. Workers are to be consulted over all aspects of the audit, including the selection of the auditor.

EMPLOYERS' ACTIVITIES AND DOCUMENTATION

Over about the past generation, health and safety regimes have been developed in industrialized countries, a good summation of which can be found in the International Labour Organization (ILO) generic Convention on Occupational Safety and Health No. 155, 1981. Elements of such regimes include the development of inter/national standards through tripartite consultations between workers, employers and governments; bipartism in the workplace, e.g., joint committees and councils; workers' rights, such as the right to refuse unsafe and unhealthy work, the right to participate, and the right to information and training; the obligation of employers to conform to a series of legislated standards, including rules governing workers' rights; and the existence of a dedicated government health and safety infrastructure, with a system of enforcement and compliance, backed by a health and safety inspectorate.

This kind of regime is now under dire threat, due to the pressures of globalization, the constraints on the powers of governments, and moves to wholesale deregulation. The most extreme manifestation of this is in moves by transnational corporations to "privatize" health and safety, to turn it into a purely internal, private affair, without pressure from governments, nor the public. Whether or not this motive is there, the fact is that corporations, especially those in the energy and chemical sectors, adopt a model which is far different from the ILO-style regime. This approach usually has four main elements:

a) responsibility for health and safety rests with management through a health and safety management system, e.g., Total Safety Management (TSM);
b) the principal method for addressing health and safety issues is through risk assessment and, in particular, Quantitative Risk Assessment (QRA);
c) risks which are identified are "managed" through techniques such as Total Loss Control; and
d) any resulting worker disabilities are subject to Disability Management through internal mechanisms such as private insurance and rehabilitation.

The theme of management runs through all of these elements. It is then only a short step to claim that all that is needed is proper management to secure health and safety. No standards or laws are required and the only right is the right to manage. Some adherents of the World Trade Organization (WTO) Agreement of 1994 see this as the avowed political aim of such globalized regimes, leaving businesses free to manage themselves properly.

Not all transnational corporations adopt these modes of health and safety management, at least on paper. Some major employers are skeptical about the value of management and auditing systems, seeing the banners proclaiming standards as well as audits and certification as a waste of time and resources. The fact that a business is certified under, say, the British standards, can tell us little about the health and safety performance of the company. We need some indication, it might be said, that the exercise is something more substantial than "paper-auditing."

Take, for example, Industry Guidance on Occupational Health and Safety (April 2001) produced by the (international) Industry Cooperation on Standards and Conformity Assessment (ICSCA) [4]. Some of the elements in this document are:

a) the adoption of an approach to enable organizations to systematically identify potential or actual job hazards; establish measurable objectives to eliminate or reduce those hazards and control any residual risks; implement programs and procedures to achieve these objectives; and, measure and check to verify performance, the effectiveness of the arrangements and to identify opportunities for continual improvement;
b) there is no prejudice in favor of risk assessment versus hazard assessment;
c) risk reduction, not risk management, is the aim of the exercise;
d) hazards and risks are best eliminated at the design and supply stage of workplaces and operations;
e) legal compliance is an important objective;
f) third-party certification is not necessary to ensure a safe and healthy workplace;
g) performance evaluation is essential, leading to corrective action; as well as
h) continuous improvement.

NATIONAL HEALTH AND SAFETY MANAGEMENT
SYSTEMS

Considering the threats to health and safety regimes world wide, the ILO Guidelines constitute, on paper, a great achievement. They appear even greater when we consider their background in national health and safety management systems, to which we will now turn.

The United Kingdom:
The British Standards Institution (BSI)

The British Standards Institution is a non-governmental standard-writing body which publishes voluntary standards. The relevant documents are: BS 8800 (1996) Guide to Occupational Health and Safety Management Systems; OHSAS 18001 (1999) Occupational Health and Safety Management Systems—Specification; and OHSAS 18002 (1999) Guidelines for the implementation of OHSAS 18001. None of these has yet been adopted as an official, certifiable BSI standard. The BS 8800 (1996) is a short document with lengthy Annexes. It does not describe a health and safety management system. Essentially, the document is a list of OHS management system elements according to whether users follow the approach of the British Health and Safety Executive (HSE) *Successful Health and Safety Management* HS(G)65 1991 (revised 1997) or BS EN ISO 14001, the environmental systems standard. The elements listed in one, the other, or both of these two approaches are: OSH policy; organizing; planning and implementation; measuring performance; audits; checking and corrective action; and management review.

Some of these are amplified in the Annexes, which include a lengthy one on risk assessment. This, as previously noted, reflects an approach to health and safety which is currently in vogue but which has no essential bearing on health and safety management, but for the fact that risk assessments are required by law in the United Kingdom (1992). (The United Kingdom does not require health and safety management systems by law, only "arrangements" to ensure the effectiveness of preventive and protective measures [The Management of Health and Safety at Work Regulations 1999, Sec. 5]).

The BS 8800 is a "performance standard" which puts forward general objectives but which sets down no essential criteria for determining whether any given system is successful, effective, or viable. The Annexes are only "informative." In particular, there are no specific elements that a health and safety audit has to incorporate, nor any definite purposes or conclusions that audits have to achieve.

The BS 8800 requires a health and safety policy which includes the organization's commitment to compliance with legal requirements as a minimum, including the legal requirement of risk assessment. However, this commitment becomes tenuous. Reviews of the system, including monitoring and measurement, are to cover compliance with OSH "arrangements," while audits refer only to "required" standards and obligations. A "compliance audit" for instance, means only compliance with a workplace health and safety policy, not compliance with the law.

Similar comments apply to the involvement of workers. The organization's OSH policy requires employee involvement and consultation; the management arrangements that the organization should make, include employee involvement, but consultation only "where appropriate." The involvement of joint health and safety committees is relegated to an Annex (B4) and this matter is raised only to downgrade the importance of committees under the heading of involvement. Continual improvement is to be part of the organization's policy and it is expressed in terms of "proactive measures;" but continual improvement is qualified by cost-effectiveness and there is no enlargement on continual improvement, even in the Annexes.

New Zealand and Australia
(AS/NZS 4801, 2000)

This standard amalgamates and supersedes two previous national standards. In its general approach it is similar to BS 8800 but there are some notable differences of emphasis. There is a commitment to comply with health and safety laws but this is only in the workplace health and safety policy and the policy is not audited, only the management system's effectiveness, e.g., in meeting the organization's policy. There is an attempt to balance the concepts of hazard and risk [5], evidently to avoid the bias toward risk assessment that characterizes BS 8800. The standard makes reference to the hierarchy of controls (hazard control methods), thus pointing to tangible improvements in workplace and working conditions; but the standard is otherwise poor on actual health and safety performance evaluation and legal compliance.

The standard is intended primarily for *external* auditing purposes. Continual improvement is part of the standard; though it is audited only to the degree that it is adopted by the organization. Like BS 8800, AS/NZS 4801 is a performance standard with all the limitations of that approach. The provisions for consulting employees and their representatives are, however, generally good.

Japan OHS-MS:
JISHA Guidelines, 1997 [6]

The Guidelines appear to have been written for the manufacturing industry, since they focus on workplace design and organization such as process design, emergency response, preventive and corrective action, and chemical safety. There is a strong emphasis on medical programs and industrial medicine.

The Japanese Guidelines are not systematic, with little coverage of management commitment, resources, and objectives. It is ironic that a country such as the

United Kingdom, with a reputation for weak and ineffectual management, should be in the forefront of management systems while a country whose manufacturing sector is reputed to be very efficiently managed, pays so little attention to management systems and their documentation. This reflects the fact that most management standards are developed by health and safety professionals who are not in the mainstream of enterprise management. It is said that they have pursued management systems as a surrogate for the sort of work that disappeared during company downsizing, when their employment contracted severely. The influence of health and safety professionals could explain the peculiarities of health and safety management documentation.

The United States

The United States does not have a national (voluntary) standard for OSH management systems. The Occupational Safety and Health Administration (OSHA) Safety and Health Program Management Guidelines (1989) are, as the title suggests, about program management, not about management *systems*. The Guidelines state that systematic management policies, procedures and practices are fundamental to the reduction of work-related injuries and illness. Employers should have a health and safety *program*, covering management commitment and employee involvement; worksite analysis; hazard prevention and control (including discipline); safety and health training; and an annual review of program effectiveness.

There was a proposal for an OSHA Safety and Health Program Rule (i.e., Regulation) in 1999, similar in many ways to the Guidelines. Like the Guidelines, the Rule would have excluded construction and agriculture. The U.S. also has its Process Management Standard, a legal requirement for hazardous workplaces such as those where there is a danger of chemical fires and explosions.

Canada

Like the United States, Canada does not have a national, voluntary standard for health and safety management systems emanating from its national standard-writing bodies. In Canada, authority over health and safety rests with the provinces and the territories, with an extensive federal (not national) jurisdiction. In several provinces, the health and safety regulatory system comes under the authority of workers' compensation boards.

Two provinces have instituted health and safety auditing systems. Alberta Partnerships in Health and Safety has instituted a Partnerships Audit (1999), a voluntary system involving external, independent audits. Employers that pass the audit get a discount on their workers' compensation premiums. Arguably, the Alberta scoring system is skewed, so that there is not enough emphasis on employers' performance evaluation, compliance, evaluation, and worker involvement, nor on systems analysis rather than employee behavior-based safety approaches. The emphasis on employee involvement is over training and worker responsibility, not on the work of joint committees.

By contrast, the Workwell Program of the Ontario Workplace Safety and Insurance Board ("enhanced" in June, 2000) is a mandatory audit instituted when an employer has a high (costly) injury rate or substandard compliance record under the Ontario OSH Act. There are no rebates for passing an audit; the system is based solely on demerits. There are quite severe penalties and remedial action required when an organization fails an audit.

Nonetheless, these auditing ventures are a possible cause for concern. It is easy to see a possible downgrading of the regulatory system so that there are virtually no enforcement measures and the regulations themselves fall into abeyance. Audits in connection with the workers' compensation system then become the surrogate for a regulatory regime, audits which are similar in nature and purpose to those in voluntary standards, written not by governments but by standard-writing bodies with loose and vague performance requirements.

THE INTERNATIONAL ORGANIZATION FOR STANDARDIZATION (ISO)

The ISO is a voluntary, standard-writing organization whose members are usually national standard-writing bodies, comprised predominantly, though not exclusively, of business people. Under the World Trade Organization (WTO) Agreement of 1994, Parties must follow international standards wherever feasible, and this includes those of ISO.

ISO Management Standards: The Background

The push toward health and safety management systems came from two main sources. The first, as has been suggested, came from the health and safety profession comprised, for instance, of industrial hygienists, auditors, and disability managers. This group saw health and safety as being enriched by management systems and benefiting from management concepts such as quality assurance, productivity, cost-benefit analysis, and continual improvement. The second source was a group in the business of quality management, that is, a group whose work was aimed at the quality of products and thus indirectly of industrial processes and production methods. The original and the most famous realization of quality management was Total Quality Management (TQM). The ISO, for instance, has produced a set of Quality Management Standards (the ISO 9000 series). The ISO then moved from Quality Management into Environmental Management (the ISO 14000 series). There was, from there, a further step toward managing workers and their work environment in the form of health and safety management standards. One strategy is to make specific references to existing quality management systems such as ISO 9000, then to address the question whether TQM and ISO 9000 principles are built into the organization's safety management system [7].

A brief look at the academic texts (which form the intellectual background of health and safety management systems) will show that in any tension between quality management and workers' health, it is always the latter that suffers the most.

One text, for instance, recommends a system of Total Safety Management (TSM) to parallel TQM [8]. Yet all the emphasis is on schemes of quality management, with a very cursory treatment of its application to health and safety. Thus Goetsch gives a series of TSM "tips" and checklists of issues, giving the impression that health and safety is really only good housekeeping. The Hierarchy of Controls, a central part of health and safety, is referred to only in passing. The treatment of toxic substances—again a prominent part of health and safety—is reduced to a 5-point checklist involving only labeling, storing, handling, and personal protective equipment! A few TSM tips are brief notes on asphyxiants, acids, and alkalis.

The academic texts tend to put an emphasis on worker behavior at the expense of health and safety systems in the workplace [9]. Now it is a part of employers' health and safety orthodoxy to place the burden of health and safety on workers rather than system changes which are usually more costly and which can exemplify a challenge to managements' right to organize work and the workplace as they see fit. But, coming from quality management, this is ironic since quality management almost always emphasizes a systems approach to quality management and control.

Safety rather than health is the prime concern, couched in the outdated terminology of "accidents" rather than traumatic injury [10]. Again employers' health and safety orthodoxy plays down the importance of disease rather than physical injury but this does not account for the emphasis on safety in quality management texts. A simpler explanation is that the authors really know very little about the discipline of health and safety, an ignorance which accords well with employer orthodoxy.

While there is reference to the cost to the organization of workplace injuries, the ethos of quality management textbooks is on employee involvement, cooperation, teamwork, and a common cause. Safety and health professionals become "catalysts, facilitators and coaches" [11]. There is a refreshing absence of the usual management incantations about the need of employees to follow the rules, with the threat of discipline when the rules are not followed. The idea of autonomous, non-hierarchical work teams was pioneered in the high-tech communications industry. In general, we can see a "flow" of quality management ideas from newer high-tech industries to more traditional industries, though the critique of employer activities (above) should warn us that most industries develop management cultures according to what they perceive to be their own business needs.

Next, the importance of legal compliance is downgraded: the "compliance mentality" is seen as detrimental to continual improvement, since the improvement stops at compliance. In all of the checklists of health and safety management topics, legal compliance is not cited. Weinstein discusses the OSHA Process Management Standard briefly but, even for those businesses which come under the Standard, compliance is not an element in audits; "compliance audit" means compliance with the company's own procedures and practices, not compliance with the law [12].

What the academic texts on quality management invariably fail to recognize is that quality management and health and safety are two different things and that they can conflict with each other. Work systems that require rapid, repetitive movements with a low degree of control over the work process mean unhealthy work. If the quality management system requires such work, then, to that extent, quality management values are inimical to worker health and well-being. It would be more candid to admit from the start that the aim of the enterprise is not the health of workers but that worker well-being in the continually improving work environment is a means to greater competitiveness. Employers in the real world sometimes recognize that the aims of quality management and of worker health are different, with only parallels of means, not ends: "Many features of effective OSH management systems are indistinguishable from those practices used to achieve quality and business excellence" [13].

ISO Management Standards: Analysis

For about the first 40 years of its existence, ISO produced only technical standards, such as equipment specifications. Though the terminology is still (misleadingly) one of "technical standards," ISO took two radically new turns, beginning in the late 1980s. The first was to produce a series of standards on Quality Management, known now as the ISO 9000 series. These standards, which include procedures for auditing, certification and registration, concern management structures and procedures, a radical departure from hardware specifications.

Quality management is, however, an established employer concern. The second big move was to produce a series of standards on Environmental Management, which is a social issue involving the public domain and heavy government regulation [14].

In 1997, a proposal was put forward to have ISO begin work on health and safety management systems, but this proposal was defeated. A second proposal was put forward but narrowly defeated in April, 2001. The latter proposal emanated largely from health and safety professionals in Great Britain, with BS 8800 put forward as the model for ISO. It is no accident that the British Guidance documents are numbered "18000", in anticipation of a new ISO 18000 health and safety management series. Such models would not have been difficult for ISO to adopt. From experience and the terms of reference for ISO 9000 and

ISO 14000, we can predict the characteristics of any ISO health and safety management system:

a) ISO management standards are not specific. A "specification standard" is one which, while voluntary and entailing no obligation to adopt it, nevertheless contains specific items. In other words, if the party adopts the standard, there are certain things it must do to conform to the standard. ISO management standards are not of this sort (in fact the terms of reference of ISO management projects prohibit such specification), nor would an ISO health and safety management standard have been any different;

b) there is no obligation to involve other parties such as workers and the public in ISO management standards. Worker involvement would probably have been even lower than in BS 8800;

c) there is no obligation to demonstrate compliance with the relevant laws and regulations. In ISO standards, the auditing of legal compliance comes about only through agreement between the employer and the auditor. This would have been no different for health and safety;

d) while ISO standards contain norms for measuring performance and standards of achievement (e.g., ISO 14031), these are not integral to the auditing procedure, nor are they an essential part of the ISO management series. Rather, the emphasis is on having management procedures in place, irrespective of outcome. ISO standards are procedural; and

e) since the only scientific technique legitimized in the WTO Agreement is risk assessment, it is highly likely that any ISO health and safety management standard would have ruled out other techniques such as hazard assessment or action based on the precautionary approach.

In all essential respects, there is every reason to believe that an ISO health and safety management standard would have been entirely different from that developed by the ILO.

CONCLUSION

If the ILO aspirations were realized in workplaces, it is arguable that health and safety management systems would be an asset to health and safety, resulting in tangible improvements in health and safety performance.

Two things have to happen. The first is that the ILO Guidelines have to be endorsed by national standard-writing centers, then translated into reality through being adopted by employers in affected workplaces. The prospects for this happening world-wide are quite good, though success will depend on how far the international labor movement and national centers are prepared to push the issue as a health and safety priority.

The second is that the WTO adopt the ILO Guidelines as the presumptive international norm or standard for health and safety management systems. It is unlikely that any Party to the WTO would put such a proposal forward and even less likely that it would be accepted. A second way this could happen is through a case in which the Guidelines were involved in a trade dispute. WTO trade tribunals would then have to decide whether the ILO Guidelines were the relevant, presumptive international standard and thus a legitimate term of trade. Such an outcome is again unlikely. Quite apart from technical arguments as to whether the ILO Guidelines constitute an "international standard" in the required sense, WTO tribunals are based on such loose and vague rules of procedure and evidence that they can decide any case on political, not judicial, grounds. Given the hostility to intervention by public institutions, it is likely that the ILO Guidelines would be given short shrift.

Overall, the degree of adoption of the ILO Guidelines and their status in the WTO will determine whether or not ISO will again enter the field and yet provide the globally accepted standard for health and safety management systems.

The implications of health and safety management systems for the practice of health and safety go much deeper than which system, if any, gets national or international recognition. One view in the labor movement is that health and safety management systems are not necessary for good health and safety practice. If we took a workplace which had a strong union and met all of the elements of the ILO-style regime, it is easy to understand the view that management systems are irrelevant to health and safety conditions in the workplace. Further, the introduction of a workplace management regime along the lines of BS 8800 would actually be counter-productive, a liability. If there is going to be a system in place, it had better be that of the ILO. The ILO Guidelines had better be adopted nationally, if only to keep out rival models. If an ILO-style scheme were introduced, it would, at worst, make little difference and, at best, formalize the procedures, recognize workers' rights, and improve conditions of work. By the same token, a management system cannot be an asset if all it does is to add one more dimension to an already unhealthy workplace.

This critique has much to commend it. But it ignores some fundamental changes that are taking place in health and safety. First, there is the point, already made, that management systems and other "voluntary standards" are being used as surrogates for regulation and all the other aspects of the ILO-style regime, including workers' rights and participation. At the same time, the regulatory authorities are changing their compliance policies in favor of "voluntary compliance," such as OSHA's Voluntary Protection Program. Even these moves belie a deeper trend. The trend among some employers is to develop their own "parallel system" of health and safety, so that they have internal or "private" regimes along the lines of those discussed above. The "external" system of regulations, requirements for workers' participation, and the role of the government inspectorate are then allowed to impinge as little as possible on management operations, e.g., by "capture" of the regulatory authorities; explicit deregulation, and the dissolution of the enforcement authority. Workers too must not be allowed to interfere with operations, and especially not by industrial disputes over health and safety, nor by collective bargaining. Such a parallel system is reflected in disability management, where a "parallel system" of private insurance and rehabilitation is used to disengage the employer from public workers' compensation provisions—the less the latter are used, the less they cost.

Internationally, the WTO Agreement has severely restricted the power of national governments to take radical measures to improve public health and safety, such as banning dangerous substances and restricting dangerous activity on any other grounds but "scientific." Science or "good science" is interpreted (entirely without rational justification) as risk assessments [15]. Governments are prohibited from taking action on grounds of public opinion, on grounds of the impact of an activity on social well-being, consumer preference or the precautionary approach; only on being able to demonstrate harm by the stringent and restrictive requirements of risk assessment. Even then, action must be the "least trade restrictive," i.e., it must disturb the status quo as little as possible. The WTO Agreement is a political barrier to effective public health and safety.

Thus it becomes important not only to insist on shoring up and developing the traditional health and safety regimes but to make health and safety once again the subject of political, industrial, and social action. The ILO-style health and safety regimes contributed indirectly to a decline in health and safety activism, as indeed, they were arguably designed to do. To allow such regimes to be dismantled and to allow employers' parallel systems to take over, would be to end up with the worst of both worlds.

Health and safety management systems have a background in theory and in various interests among employers and workplace health and safety professionals. These have resulted in a number of national systems emanating from national standard-writing centers and from employers' organizations. In some cases these systems have been recognized as national standards. The contenders for an international standard have been the International Organization of Standardization (ISO) and the International Labour Organization (ILO). The quality and environmental management systems of ISO indicate what an ISO health and safety management standard would look like. The ILO Guidelines on Safety and Health Management Systems, by contrast, are stringent, specific, and potentially effective in improving health and safety performance in the workplace.

ACKNOWLEDGMENTS

For advice and information on national systems, the author is grateful to Kevin Flaherty (AFL-CLC, Canada); Bjorn Erikson (LO, Norway); Anna Prambourg (TCO, Sweden); Tom Mellish and Owen Tudor (TUC, Great Britain); Erik Greenslade (NZCTU, New Zealand); and Bill Kojola (AFL-CIO, USA). For labor perspectives on health and safety management systems, the author is indebted to Bill Chedore (CLC, Canada) and Cathy Walker (CAW, Canada). The author thanks Tom Ott (Motorola, USA) for information on employers' perspectives.

REFERENCES

1. The tripartite Meeting of Experts which finalized the Guidelines at the ILO in Geneva in April 2001 was chaired by Dr. K.E. Poppendick (German Government). The three groups consisted of seven persons each. The spokesperson of the government group was Dr. D. Podgorski (Poland); the spokesperson of the workers' group was Dr. D. Bennett (Canada); and the spokesperson of the employers' group was Dr. J. Asherson (U.K.). There were also observers from international organizations concerned with health and management.
2. Cathy Walker, CAW (Canada), personal communication.
3. Leading critiques of risk assessment are Ginsburg R.: "Quantitative Risk Assessment and the Illusion of Safety," *New Solutions, 3*:2, Winter 1993; O'Brien M., *Making Better Environmental Decisions, An Alternative to Risk Assessment,* Part I, What Is Wrong With Risk Assessment? MIT, Cambridge, 2000; and "Trading Away Public Health: WTO Obstacles to Effective Toxics Controls," *Journal of Public Health Policy, 21*:3, 2000.
4. Members of this group are mainly transnational corporations in the high tech and industrial manufacturing sectors, though a few of the 120 members are petrochemical companies.
5. In the *ILO Guidelines on Occupational Safety and Health Management Systems* (2001), there are balanced definitions of hazard and hazard assessment, risk and risk assessment.
6. "Occupational Health and Safety Management Systems: Review and Analysis of International, National and Regional Systems; and Proposals For a New International Document," ILO, Geneva, 1998, pages 76-77.
7. Weinstein, M. B., *Total Quality Safety Management and Auditing.* Boca Raton: New York, 1997.
8. Goetsch, D. L., *Implementing Total Safety Management: Safety, Health and Competitiveness in the Global Marketplace.* New Jersey: Prentice Hall, 1998.
9. Nichols, T. and Tucker, E., *Occupational Health and Safety Management Systems in the U.K. and Ontario, Canada: A Political Economy Perspective,* North York, Canada: 1999, page 20; also Weinstein, op cit., pages 183-190.
10. Nichols, T., and Tucker, E., op cit page 21; Weinstein op cit. pages 3-5.
11. Goetsch, D. L., op cit., page (iii).
12. Weinstein, M. B., op cit., pages 178-179.
13. *Industry Guide,* op cit, page 1.
14. Evidence as to the reasons for ISO's radical change in direction are anecdotal. One story is that the German employers wished to produce a standard which, in international trade law, would supersede regional and national standards such as the European Environmental Management and Audit System (EMAS). Some employer groups opposed ISO getting into environmental management on the grounds that environmental protection was a social issue and not primarily one of business management; the same arguments apply to health and safety management standards.

For arguments that EMAS is more stringent and effective than ISO 14000, see Tickner, J.: "ISO 14000: Will It Deter Cleaner Production?," *New Solutions, 8*:3, 1998. For a political critique of ISO management standards, see Bennett, D. "Beware ISO," *New Solutions, 7*:3, Spring 1997.

15. See the WTO Agreement on the Application of Sanitary and Phytosanitary Measures and the Agreement on Technical Barriers to Trade (which are components of the WTO Agreement 1994); also NAFTA, comparable chapters and Chapter II, Investment.

Index

Academic freedom and the independence
  of research, 130-131
Agriculture and debate over using
  pesticides, 97-98
Alar, 57, 104
ALARA principle and radiation exposure,
  40-42, 51
Alberta Partnerships in Health and Safety,
  176-177
American Association for Cancer
  Research (AACR), 103
American Cancer Society (ACS), 111,
  112, 117
American Conference of Governmental
  Industrial Hygienists (ACGIH),
  43-47, 51-52
American Industrial Health Council
  (AHIC), 107
Ames, Bruce N., 104, 106, 115
Anastasias, Paul T., 139
Animal testing, cancer and, 105-106
Asbestos, 45, 119-120
Audits and ILO guidelines on
  safety/health management systems,
  172
Australia, 175
Austria, 98
Auto industry and cleanup strategy, 69
Ayres, Raymond, 145

Bans and phase-outs, chemical, 71,
  136-137
Barry Commoner, 135
Belanger, Jean, 20

Benyus, Janie, 139, 145
Big Green in California, 57, 58
Bioaccumulation factor (BCF), 62
Bio-based materials, 138-139
Biomimicry, 143
Biomimicry (Benyus), 139
Biosafety protocol and genetically
  modified organisms, 166
Bis-phenol A (BPA), 5
Black, Jim, 24
Bouchard, Robert, 20-21
Boulding, Kenneth, 138
Bovine growth hormone (BGH), 117
Britain, 30-31, 112, 174-176
British Health and Safety Executive
  (HSE), 174
British Standards Institution, 174-175
Brundtland Commission (1987), 9
Burrows, Mae, 32
Business community/operations, 8, 79,
  126, 144-145
  See also International Labor
    Organization; International
    Organization for Standardization;
    Prevention, Pollution; Safety/Health
    Management Systems, ILO's
    Guidelines on; Workplace
    Hazardous Materials Information
    System

Canada and national safety/health
  management systems, 176-177
  See also individual subject headings
Canada Labour Code, 22

Canada-U.S. Free Trade Agreement (FTA), 115
Canadian Auto Workers (CAW), 25
Canadian Cancer Society (CCS), 9, 122
Canadian Chemical Producers' Association (CCPA), 2-3, 20
Canadian Farmworkers' Union (CPU), 57
Canadian Labour Congress (CLC)
  alliances with national/regional environmental organizations, 9
  cancer prevention, 9, 123
  Environment Committee, 67
  International Confederation of Free Trade Unions, 11
  Just Transition for Workers During Environmental Change, 34, 91
  pesticides, 57-59, 62
  prevention, pollution, 3
  taxation system on businesses using toxic chemicals, 8
  toxics use reduction, 8
  Workplace Hazardous Materials Information System, 2
  Workplace Health and Safety Committee, 67
  See also Labour and the environment at the CLC; Pollution prevention strategy, the CLC's; individual subject headings
Canadian Manufacturers' Association (CMA), 20
Canadian Standards Association, 12, 50, 150-151
Canadian Strategy for Cancer Control (CSCC), 123
Canadian Union of Public Employees (CUPE), 34
Cancer Battles and the Sleep of Reason
  experts, why should policymakers consult the, 102-107
  hazards, occupational: a case study, 107-108
  pesticides, 97-98
  risk assessment is not only science of environmental health, 98-102
  See also Politics of Cancer Revisited; Secret History of the War on Cancer

Cancer-Gate (Epstein)
  Canadian moves toward cancer prevention, 122-124
  collapse of federal/governmental initiatives, 118-119
  Epstein's previous books, 117
  limitations of book, 118
  precautionary principle, 119-121
  toxics use reduction, 120-121
Cancer prevention and CLC, 9, 123
Capitalism, natural, 141-145
Capture as a pollution control method, 68, 86
Carbon-based computing, 139
Carcinogeneticists as experts used in policymaking, 103, 104
Carson, Rachel L., 141
Cartahena Protocol to the UN Convention on Biodiversity in 1992, 166
Castleman, B., 46
Cell phones and cancer, 132
Chedore, Bill, 183
Chemical Engineering Process, 73
Chemical hazards
  bans and phase-outs, 71, 136-137
  Canadian Environmental Protection Act of 1988, 1, 4-5
  Globally Harmonized System for Chemical Classification and Labeling, 12
  hazard vs. risk assessment, 12
  rights, workers' environmental, 17-19, 25, 31, 74-76, 153, 170-171
  substitution, chemical, 89, 121-122
  users vs. producers, 3, 5, 121
  See also Pesticides; Pollution prevention strategy, the CLC's; Prevention, pollution; Toxics Use Reduction; Workplace Hazardous Materials Information System
Chemicals, Work and Cancer, 107
Clapp, Richard W., 116
CLC. See Canadian Labour Congress
Cleanup strategy, 69
Closed-loop process/systems, 72, 89
Codex Alimentarius Commission, 154

Collaborative on Health and the Environment, 132

Cominco smelter complex, 69

Committees on Occupational Safety and Health (COSH) in the U.S., 30-31

Commoner, Barry, 87-88, 140

Communication, Energy and Paperworkers' Union (CEP), 34, 89

Confidentiality, de facto business, 126

Connell, Brian, 20

Constitution, Canadian, 6

Control from prevention, distinguishing pollution, 3, 5, 47-51, 68-69, 83-89

Cook, Doug, 20

Coronado, Rick, 32

COSH Committees (Committees on Occupational Safety and Health) in the U.S., 30-31

Daly, Herman, 9, 145

Daniels, Mark, 20

Daubert case (1993), 131

Davis, Devra, 9, 125

Dawes, David, 21

Deep ecology, 141, 145

Dehavilland, 25

De-industrialization and the decay of productive industries, 69

Dematerilization and a sustainable materials policy, 140

Deregulation movement and health/safety management, 172-173

Destruction as a pollution control method, 86

Detoxification and a sustainable materials policy, 140

Diamond, Bob, 32

Diet and cancer, 108, 129, 130

Dilution as a pollution control method, 68, 86

Disaster Capitalism (Klein), 130

Dissolution as a pollution control method, 86

Doll, Richard, 106, 129

Doubt, cancer secrecy and the manufacture of, 127-128

Duplication in area of environmental protection, 7

Ecology of commerce, 141-145

Ecology of Commerce (Hawken), 145

Economics and environmental protection, 69-70, 141-145

Education, public/worker, 21-22, 118, 130

Electro-magnetic field (EMF), 132

Elimination of pollutants, virtual, 71-72, 89

Emanuel, Ezekiel J., 129

Emission controls, pollutant, 85

Employer requirements as an element of CLC's pollution strategy, 76-77

End-point *vs.* science-driven health policy, 132

Energy and Chemical Workers Union (ECWU), 34

Engineered materials, 138

Engineering as key to occupational health, 53-54

England, 30-31, 112, 174-176

Environmental Cancer-A Political Disease? (Lichter & Rothman). *See Cancer Battles and the Sleep of Reason*

Environmental Committee, CLC's, 31-35, 67

Environmental non-governmental organizations (ENGOs), 157-158

Environmental Protection Agency (EPA), 46, 111

Environmental theory, 141-142

Epidemiologists as experts used in policymaking, 103-104

Epstein, Samuel, 9, 106, 117, 130

See also Cancer *listings*

Erikson, Bjorn, 182

Evanoff, S. P., 73

Evaporation as a pollution control method, 68, 86

Experts' role in environmental health policy-making. *See Cancer Battles and the Sleep of Reason*

Exxon, 20

Fast Food Nation (Schlosser), 130
Fats and cancer, dietary, 108
Filtration as a pollution control method, 68, 86
Fire Brigades' Union (FBU), 30
Flaherty, Kevin, 182
Food and Drug Administration (FDA), 111
Forest issues, 33, 156-158
Forest Stewardship Council (FSC), 157

Galbraith, John K., 138
Galland, Adolf, 106
GATT. *See* General Agreement on Tariffs and Trade
Geiser, Kenneth, 135-140
General Agreement on Tariffs and Trade (GATT) in 1994, 150, 154, 157, 158
Genetically modified organisms (GMOs), 166
German Democratic Republic (GDR), 98
Globalization and subordination of national regulations, 11-12, 115-116, 167, 172-173
See also individual subject headings
Globally Harmonized System for Chemical Classification and Labeling (GHS), 12
Goulet, Diane, 34
Great Britain, 30-31, 112, 174-176
Great Lakes, 4
Greene, Gayle, 129
Green Job Creation, 10. 34
Greenslade, Erik, 182

Hawken, Paul, 130, 138, 144
Hazardous Materials Information Review Commission (HMIRC), 24, 25
"Hazardous Waste Reduction in the Aerospace Industry" (Evanoff), 73
Hazards of Work, The, 107
Hazard *vs.* risk assessment, 12, 88-89, 98-102, 171, 180
Health-Based Exposure Limits (HBELs), 46

Health/safety management, workplace
Canadian Standards Association, 12, 50
International Labor Organization, 31, 47-52
International Organization for Standardization, 12, 150, 158-160, 167, 177-180
labour and the environment at the CLC, 30-31
See also Occupational health/environment issues; Safety/Health Management Systems, ILO's Guidelines on
Higginson, John, 106
History of Cancer Control in the United States, 1946-1971, 127
Horton, Richard, 129
Hydrogenase used to produce hydrogen, 139
Hygiene *vs.* medicine, prevention and industrial, 84-85
Hypercar, 144

ILO. *See* International Labor Organization
Imperial Oil, 20
Industry Cooperation on Standards and Conformity Assessment (ICSCA), 173
Integrated Pest Management (IPM), 12
Interest group liberalism, 57, 58
International Agency for Research on Cancer (IARC), 105, 123, 129
International Commission on Radiological Protection (ICRP), 39, 40-43, 52
International Confederation of Free Trade Unions (ICFTU), 11, 13, 91, 159, 163-167
International Congress of Scientific and Social Campaign Against Cancer (1936), 127
International Electrotechnical Commission, 149
International Journal of Health Services, 118

International Labor Organization (ILO)
  Convention on Occupational Health
    Services, 5
  health/safety management, workplace,
    31, 47-52
  International Commission on
    Radiological Protection, 40
  International Confederation of Free
    Trade Unions, 11
  Occupational Health and Safety
    Convention of 1981, 159, 172
  prevention, pollution, 89
  Saskatchewan Law of 1972, 18
  See also Safety/Health Management
    Systems, ILO's Guidelines on
International Organization for Standardi-
    zation (ISO)
  application of, 155-156
  complicating factors, 157-158
  health/safety management, workplace,
    12, 150, 158-160, 167, 177-180, 182
  history of, 149-150
  ILO's safety/health management
    system guidelines, 167, 177-180,
    182
  International Confederation of Free
    Trade Unions, report to the, 163-167
  ISONET, 154
  national standards bodies, 12, 150-152
  prevention, pollution, 87
  sectoral standards, 156-157
  14000 Series on Environmental
    Management, 150, 153-159,
    164-166, 180
  18000 Series on Health and Safety,
    150, 179
  9000 Series on Quality Management,
    149-150, 152-153, 164-165,
    177-180
  summary/conclusions, 160
  World Trade Organization, 157, 180
International Woodworkers of America
    (IWA-Canada), 32
Interstate Commerce Clause, U.S., 6
ISO. See International Organization for
    Standardization
Issue management, 128-129

Japan, 175-176
Jolley, Linda, 21, 22
Jurisdiction over the environment, 7-8, 78
Just Transition for Workers During
    Environmental Change, 10, 34-35,
    90-92, 144

Klein, Naomi, 130
Knote, Helga, 32
Know about chemical hazards, the right
    to, 17-19, 25, 31, 75-76, 118
  See also Workplace Hazardous
    Materials Information System
Kohler, Brian, 34
Kojola, Bill, 182
Kyoto Protocol, 34-35

Labeling provisions/standards, 21, 22, 25,
    165-166
Labour and the environment at the CLC:
    story of the convergence
  academics alienated from the union
    fraternity, 29
  Britain and Canada, differences
    between, 30-31
  Environment Committee, 31-35
  union staff numbers and ratio of staff to
    rank-and-file members, 29
Law reform and cancer secrecy, 131-132
Lead, airborne, 88
Legal compliance and guidelines on
    safety/health management systems,
    171, 179
Legislation
  British North America Act of 1867,
    6, 7
  Canadian Environmental Protection
    Act (CEPA) of 1988, 1, 4-5, 8, 74,
    77, 123, 155
  Clean Air Acts, 77-78
  Constitution Act of 1981, 6, 7
  Hazardous Products Act, 24
  Occupational Health and Safety Acts,
    76
  Pest Control Products Act (PCPA), 59

[Legislation]
Pest Control Products Regulations Act (PCPR), 59
Saskatchewan Law of 1972, 18, 23
Species at Risk Act, 33
(U.K.) Health and Safety at Work Act, 18
(U.S.) Clean Air Act, 58, 78
(U.S.) Delaney amendment (1958) to Food, Drugs and Cosmetic Act, 116
(U.S.) Massachusetts Toxics Use Reduction Act of 1989, 6, 88, 121-123
(U.S.) New Jersey Pollution Prevention Act of 1991, 88
(U.S.) Occupational Safety and Health Act, 18
(U.S.) Pollution Prevention Act of 1990, 88
Lethal Concentration (LC), 22, 61-62
Lethal Dose (LD), 22, 61-62
Lichter, S. Robert, 97
  See also Cancer Battles and the Sleep of Reason
Lifestyle and cancer, 130
Lloyd, Gordon, 20
Lowell Center for Sustainable Production, 140

Marsh, George P., 142
Martin, Dick, 33
Marxist theory, 143
Massachusetts toxics use reduction program, 73
Material safety data sheets (MSDSs), 21-26, 74, 75-76, 126
Materials Matter (Geiser), 135-140
Maximum Residue Limits (MRLs), 12, 113
Mazankowski, Don, 57
Mazzocchi, Tony, 34
McDonnell Douglas, 25
Media-shift as a pollution control method, 86
Medical profession in occupational health disciplines, 50-51

Medicine *vs.* hygiene, prevention and industrial, 84-85
Mellish, Tom, 182
Mercier, Richard, 20
Mercury in surface waters, 88
Merrill, Michael, 91-92
Minimization strategy for workplace hazards, 52
Minnesota, 121
Mirer, Franklin, 22
MOE system, 99-101
MTBE, 5
Multicausality axiom, 113
Multilateral Agreement on Investment (MAI), 167

Nader, Ralph, 107
National Cancer Institute (NCI), 111, 112, 117, 127
National standards bodies, 12, 150-152, 174-177, 180
Natural Capitalism (Hawken, Lovins, & Lovins), 130, 141-145
Natural medicine, 130
Nature, modeling materials and their uses on the processes of, 137-138
Neutralization as a pollution control method, 68
New Jersey, 121
New Republic, 129
New York Review of Books, 129
New Zealand, 175
Nitrogen oxide, 58
"No Pollution Prevention Without Income Protection" (Merrill), 91-92
North American Free Trade Agreement (NAFTA), 11, 12, 115, 116, 154, 157

Obesity and cancer, 129
Occupational Health and Safety Convention of 1981, 159, 172
Occupational health/environment issues
American Conference of Governmental Industrial Hygienists, 43-47

[Occupational health/environment issues]
  Canadian record on, 13
  cancer, 107-108
  engineering as key to occupational
    health, 53-54
  International Commission on
    Radiological Protection, 40-43
  International Labor Organization, 31,
    47-52
  overview, 39-40
  scientific practitioners and social
    issues, relationship between, 39
  summary/conclusions, 51-54
  See also Health/safety management,
    workplace; Pollution prevention
    strategy, the CLC's; Prevention,
    pollution; Safety/Health
    Management Systems, ILO's
    Guidelines on
Occupational Safety and Health Adminis-
    tration (OSHA), 17, 107, 111
Oil, Chemical and Atomic Workers
    (OCAW), 34, 89
Oregon, 121
Organization for Economic Cooperation
    and Development (OECD), 91, 105
Ott, Tom, 183

Paint stripping, process reformulation in,
    73
Partiality and cancer research
    findings/results, 128
Participate, workers' right to, 31, 74, 171
Performance standards, 48, 171
Personal protective equipment (PPE), 84
Pesticides
  Cancer Battles and the Sleep of
    Reason, 97-98
  cleanup strategy, 69
  cosmetic use of, banning the, 6
  registration process, review of, 57-63
  risk vs. hazard assessment, 12
  secrets, trade, 21
  Workplace Hazardous Materials
    Information System, 25-26
Peto, Richard, 106

Photozyme used to manufacture vitamin
    C, 139
Policy-making, environmental health. See
    Cancer listings
Politics of Cancer, The (Epstein), 111,
    117, 119, 130
Politics of Cancer Revisited, The
    (Epstein)
  disappointment with, 117
  globalization, 115-116
  outline of, 111-112
  perspectives on environmental cancer,
    compendium of, 112
  Politics of Cancer, update on The, 111
  regulatory programs, establishment
    theory opposing, 113-115
  theory of environmental cancer,
    112-113
Pollution prevention strategy, the CLC's
  aim of, 6
  business community, 79
  Canada's unwillingness to create
    effective legislation, 77
  control and prevention, distinction
    between, 68-69
  employers required to produce
    pollution prevention/control
    programs, 76-77
  jurisdiction over the environment,
    7-8, 78
  main elements, strategy has four,
    71-77
  objections to, environmentalists', 8
  obstacles, 77-79
  outside pollution, workplace pollution
    treated equally with, 70
  primacy of prevention, 67-69
  socioeconomic effects of pollution
    prevention measures, 69-70
  toxics use reduction, 72-74
  understood, not well, 8
  workers' environmental rights, 74-75
  zero discharge, 71-72, 76
  See also Prevention, pollution
Port Alberni pulp mill, 69, 70
Pragmatic limits vs. industrial hygiene
    with no limits, 46

Prambourg, Anna, 182
Precautionary principle, 119-121
Precipitation as a pollution control
    method, 68, 86
"Prevent Cancer Now!," 9
Prevention, pollution
    Canadian Labour Congress, 3
    Constitution, Canadian, 7
    control distinguished from, 3, 5, 47-51,
        68-69, 83-89
    defining terms, 83
    Hierarchy of Prevention and Controls,
        89, 90
    International Organization for
        Standardization, 87
    Just Transition for Workers During
        Environmental Change, 90-92
    pesticides, banning/restricting
        nonagricultural use of, 6
    primary, 50-51, 84-85
    revolt leading to more focus on,
        87-89
    secondary, 50-51, 84-85
    Superfund for Workers, 89-90
    tertiary, 50-51, 84-85
    See also Cancer listings; Pollution
        prevention strategy, the CLC's;
        Toxics Use Reduction
Primary prevention, 50-51, 84-85
Privatization movement and health/safety
    management, 172-173
Process and Production Methods (PPMs),
    165, 166
Producers vs. users, chemical, 3, 5, 121
Proposed Regulatory Decision Document
    (PRDD), 60
Public Health Agency of Canada, 123
Pulp mills, 69, 70

Quality management and the ISO,
    149-150, 152-153, 164-165, 177-180

Radiation exposure limits, 40-43
Radioactive fallout, 88
Rappaport, S. M., 43

REACH (Registration, Evaluation, and
    Authorization of Chemicals)
    program, EU's, 117, 118, 120-122
Reactive vs. precautionary approach, 120
Reagan, Ronald, 79
Recycling and reuse of materials, 138
Recycling as a pollution control method,
    out-of-process, 68, 86
Refuse unsafe work, right to, 18, 25, 31,
    75
Regulatory programs, cancer
    establishment theory opposing,
    113-115
Remedial vs. prevention/control services,
    50-51
Renewable materials, 138
Research findings, control/suppression of,
    127, 128, 130-131
Resource productivity, radically
    increased, 142-143
Rights, workers' environmental, 17-19,
    25, 31, 74-76, 118, 153, 170-171
Rio Declaration of 1992, 119, 142
Risk vs. hazard assessment, 12, 88-89,
    98-102, 171, 180
Roach, S. A., 43
Rosenberg, Maurice, 19
Rothman, Stanley, 97
    See also Cancer Battles and the Sleep
        of Reason

Safety/Health Management Systems,
    ILO's Guidelines on
    employers' activities and
        documentation, 172-173
    history of the ILO, 169
    International Organization for
        Standardization, 167, 177-180, 182
    Japan, 175-176
    national safety/health management
        systems, 174-177, 180
    New Zealand and Australia, 175
    summary/conclusions, 180-182
    three parts, guidelines are in, 170
    United Kingdom, 174-175
    United States, 176

[Safety/Health Management Systems, ILO's Guidelines on]
  voluntary acceptance of ILO instruments, 169-170
  workers' rights/perspectives/experiences, 170
  World Trade Organization, 180-182
  See also Health/safety management, workplace; Occupational health/environment issues
Sass, Bob, 18, 31
Schlosser, Eric, 130
Science, health policy in relation to, 132
Scientific constituency, recognizing the voice of the, 52-53
Secondary prevention, 50-51, 84-85
Second Law of Thermodynamics, 10
Secret History of the War on Cancer, The (Davis)
  academic freedom and the independence of research, 130-131
  availability of cancer studies, lack of, 127
  business confidentiality, de facto, 126
  carcinogens examined for their significance in the war on cancer, 126
  communicating campaigns to the public, 130
  doubt, the manufacture of, 127-128
  law reform, 131-132
  literary social history, 125-126
  modes of secrecy, 126-127
  reception of book, 129-130
  research findings, control/suppression of, 127, 128
  science, health policy in relation to, 132
  social costs of cancer care, 132
  systematic analysis, lack of, 125
  trade secrecy and proprietary information, 126
  two aspects to the question of fighting cancer, 125
Secret protection, trade, 21, 22-24, 126

Sectoral standards and the ISO, 156-157
Selikoff, Irving, 106
Service-flow model and natural capitalism, 143, 144
Shaw, George B., 108
Silent Spring (Carson), 141, 145
Simon, John, 137
Social costs of cancer care, 132
Social ecology, 141
Social justice, 144
Social movements and moving from the local to the national, 11
Socioeconomic effects of pollution prevention measures, 69-70
Specification standards, 48, 171, 180
Stainsby, Cliff, 34
Stallones, R., 107
Standards *vs.* rights, 17-19
State-changes as a pollution control method, 86
Steady-State Economics (Daly), 145
Stockholm Declaration of 1972, 142
Substitution, chemical, 89, 121-122
Substitution analysis, 99
Successful Health and Safety Management, 174
Sunsetting/sunrising chemicals, 71
Superfund for Workers, 89-90
Supreme Court, U.S., 131
Sustainability, 9-10
  See also Materials Matter; Natural capitalism
Sweden, 98

Tarlau, Eileen S., 46
Taxation system on businesses using toxic chemicals, 8
Technical Barriers to Trade (TBT), GATT Agreement on, 154, 158
Teitelbaum, Daniel, 127
Tertiary prevention, 50-51, 84-85
Thatcher, Margaret, 79
Theories on environmental cancer, 112-113
Theory, environmental, 141-142
Thermodynamics, Second Law of, 10

Threshold Limit Values (TLVs), 43-47, 51-52
Tobacco, 104, 129
Total quality management (TQM), 153, 177-178
Total Safety Management (TSM), 178
Toxics Use Reduction (TUR)
  Cancer-Gate, 120-121
  CLC making progress in, 8
  detoxification and a sustainable materials policy, 140
  Massachusetts Toxics Use Reduction Act of 1989, 6, 88, 121-123
  Merrill, Michael, 92
  objections to, environmentalists', 8
  outside pollution, workplace pollution treated equally with, 70
  pesticides, 59
  pollution prevention strategy, the CLC's, 72-74
Trade secret protection, 21, 22-24, 126
Trade Union Advisory Council (TUAC), 91
Tudor, Owen, 182

United Auto Workers (UAW), 32
United Kingdom, 30-31, 112, 174-176
United Nations
  Conference on Environment and Development (1992), 150
  Convention on Biodiversity in 1992, Cartahena Protocol to the, 166
  scientific constituency, recognizing the voice of the, 52-53
  World Commission on Environment and Development (1987), 9
  See also International Labor Organization
United States and national safety/health management systems, 176
United Steelworkers (USW), 34
Updike, John, 10
U.S. National Safety Council, 84
Users vs. producers, chemical, 3, 5, 121
Utilization as a pollution control method, 68

Vagueness in area of environmental protection, 7
Video display terminals (VDTs) and cancer, 132
Virtual elimination of pollutants, 71-72
Vitamin C, photozyme used to manufacture, 139

Walker, Cathy, 26-27, 183
Warner, John C., 139
Whate, Rich, 26
Whistle-blower protection, 74-75
Wingspread version of the precautionary approach, 120
Woodcock, Loretta, 32
Work Can Be Dangerous to Your Health, 107
Work environment. See Occupational health/environment issues
Workers' environmental rights, 17-19, 25, 31, 74-76, 118, 153, 170-171
Workplace Hazardous Materials Information System (WHMIS)
  Bouchard (Robert) and Jolley (Linda) keep project on track, 20-21
  Canadian Chemical Producers' Association, 2-3
  educating workers and labeling/data sheets, 21-22
  implementation and enforcement, 24-26
  material safety data sheets, 21-26, 75-76
  pollution prevention strategy, the CLC's, 77
  tensions within/between three constituencies involved in, 19-20
  trade secret protection, 21, 22-24
  tripartite structure of the project, 19
Workwell Program of the Ontario Workplace Safety and Insurance Board, 177
World Health Organization (WHO), 140

World Trade Organization (WTO)
Agreement of 1994, 177
Cartahena Protocol to the UN
Convention on Biodiversity in 1992,
166
globalization, facilitating, 11, 115-116,
167
ILO guidelines on safety/health
management systems, 180-182
International Confederation of Free
Trade Unions, report to the,
163-164

[World Trade Organization (WTO)]
International Organization for Standardization, 157, 180
national standards, requirements for, 12
Wynn, Tom, 32

Yaeger, Chuck, 106

Zero discharge as an element of CLC's
pollution strategy, 71-72, 76
Zero Waste, 139
Ziem, G., 46

In Praise

In *Northern Exposures*, David Bennett offers an important contribution to the contemporary history of the Canadian labor and environmental movements. His well-argued analysis chronicles the labor movement's shift from a narrow focus on occupational health to a much broader conceptualization of hazard prevention. The analysis is well-grounded in the legal and constitutional history of the period, and it also offers rich insights into the political struggles between the business and labor communities and the strategic struggles within the labor and environmental movements. If we are going to effectively advance an international movement for a sustainable future, we need critical retrospectives such as this on the efforts that have brought us major steps forward.

Ken Geiser, Ph.D.
Professor of Work Environment
Co-Director, Lowell Center for Sustainable Production
University of Massachusetts Lowell

Northern Exposures is a unique and valuable book. David Bennett writes as someone who, for more than 20 years, was in the forefront of the Canadian labor movement's struggles for a safer workplace and healthier environment. Based on his participation in numerous domestic and international negotiations, he provides not only a valuable historical account of those struggles but also a keen analytical treatment—reflecting his academic training as a philosopher—of many controversies in Canadian environmental policy. We do not have nearly enough high-quality studies on the interface of science and public policy, and Dr. Bennett's book is a powerful antidote to the contemporary tendency to depoliticize conflicts over underlying values through the jargon of "risk management."

Ted Schrecker
Associate Professor, Department of Epidemiology and
Community Medicine
Principal Scientist, Institute of Population Health
University of Ottawa

A SELECTION OF TITLES FROM THE
WORK, HEALTH AND ENVIRONMENT SERIES
Series Editors, *Charles Levenstein, Robert Forrant and John Wooding*

AT THE POINT OF PRODUCTION
The Social Analysis of Occupational
and Environmental Health
Edited by Charles Levenstein

BEYOND CHILD'S PLAY
Sustainable Product Design in the
Global Doll-Making Industry
Sally Edwards

ENVIRONMENTAL UNIONS
Labor and the Superfund
Craig Slatin

METAL FATIGUE
American Bosch and the Demise
of Metalworking in the Connecticut River Valley
Robert Forrant

SHOES, GLUES AND HOMEWORK
Dangerous Work in the Global Footwear Industry
Pia Markkanen

WITHIN REACH?
Managing Chemical Risks in Small Enterprises
David Walters

INSIDE AND OUT
Universities and Education for Sustainable Development
Edited by Robert Forrant and Linda Silka

WORKING DISASTERS
The Politics of Recognition and Response
Edited by Eric Tucker

LABOR-ENVIRONMENTAL COALITIONS
Lessons from a Louisiana Petrochemical Region
Thomas Estabrook

CORPORATE SOCIAL RESPONSIBILITY
FAILURES IN THE OIL INDUSTRY
Edited by Charles Woolfson and Matthias Beck